Orthopedics of the Upper and Lower Limb

K. Mohan Iyer
Editor

Orthopedics of the Upper and Lower Limb

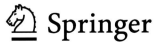 Springer

Editor
Dr. K. Mohan Iyer
Bangalore University
Bangalore
Karnataka
India

ISBN 978-1-4471-4446-5   ISBN 978-1-4471-4447-2   (eBook)
DOI 10.1007/978-1-4471-4447-2
Springer London Heidelberg New York Dordrecht

Library of Congress Control Number: 2012948544

Printed on acid-free paper

Springer is part of Springer Science+Business Media (www.springer.com)

Dedicated to my wife,
Nalini K. Mohan
And
Daughter, Dr. Deepa Iyer
M.B.,B.S.,MRCP(UK)
And
Son, Mr. Rohit Iyer, B.E.

Foreword

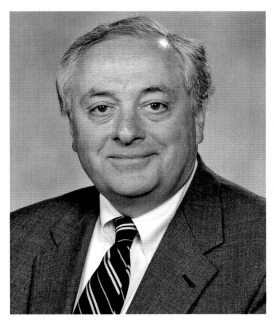

Several decades ago I was fortunate to hear Dr. Iyer speak about a limited, posterior greater trochanteric osteotomy as an adjunct to a posterior approach to the hip. Since then I have used this method, as it allows easy access to the hip for joint replacement and then a secure posterior capsule and short external rotator muscle repair upon joint closure. Postoperative dislocations ceased to be an issue. As you might recognize, I have looked forward to additional contributions from Dr. Iyer, and here we have it – General Principles of Orthopedics and Trauma, Orthopedics of the Upper and Lower Limb and Trauma management in Orthopedics (Springer).

What a huge task to organize such books: Deciding on the material to be included, writing multiple chapters, and asking for skilled contributors who will embrace the challenge and have the talents to write either a general or subspecialty chapter. The text is aimed at the newcomer to this field of medicine, and it will serve that purpose quite well. I have always felt the best approach to learning orthopedic surgery is to read, cover to cover, a text such as this, aggressively study anatomy, read about the problems in the patients under one's care, read subspecialty texts, and read at least the abstracts in selected journals. By doing these things one can be an educated person in the field – but it starts with the basic text!

In addition to the fundamentals, Dr. Iyer has added details about trauma and regional orthopedics. A cad has said only two types of doctors are necessary, and the others are optional. One of these is a physician who cares for broken bones. Details about fractures are essential to the field and to humanistic patient care. The regional chapters serve as a transition to the later reading about each anatomic region in detail, what will be required to become an orthopedic surgeon.

So there you have it. An editor who is an energetic, dedicated scholar and teacher. Plus, the type of textbook most needed to jump into the field of musculoskeletal medicine and surgery. Learning is a joy. Lucky readers, enjoy the intellectual journey.

Rochester, MN, USA   Robert H. Cofield, M.D.

Preface

This book is mainly an introduction to the principles of Orthopedics, which is written by different Orthopedic Surgeons, who have specialized in the subjects they have written in. This volume details various Orthopedic conditions (other than trauma) by regions in the upper and lower limb.

I was an undergraduate and post-graduate teacher at the University of Liverpool, UK, and the University of London, UK, for the undergraduates and for the final FRCS candidates. On returning home to Bangalore, India, I was an undergraduate teacher at St. John's Hospital, Bangalore, India, and at M.S. Ramaiah Medical Teaching Hospital, Bangalore, India, and I am indebted to all my students for their constant desire to master Orthopedics at their young age. Above all, I would like to thank all my teachers who did not spare any effort to discuss with me topics of Orthopedic interest, both in the lecture hall and in their spare time.

I am deeply indebted to my dear friend, Mr. Magdi E. Greiss, M.D., M.Ch. (Orth), FRCS, Senior Consultant Orthopedic Surgeon North Cumbria University Hospitals, UK, Former President, BOFAS, UK, for his timely help in specially preparing the snaps that have been used in this book, despite him being extremely busy in setting up of a foot and ankle clinic for the World Orthopaedic Concern in developing countries.

I would express my sincere thanks to Mr. Adhish Avasthi, M.B.B.S., M.S. Orth., MRCS Registrar Orthopedics and Mr. Richard Hill, M.B. Ch.B., FRCS Ed, FRCS (Tr & Orth) Ed, Consultant Orthopedic Surgeon, Department of Trauma & Orthopedics, St Richard's Hospital, Chichester PO19 6SE, West Sussex, UK, for his comprehensive description on Common Sports Injuries, which is a subspeciality in vogue at the moment. I would also like to thank Dr. Suhas Namjoshi, Consultant Radiologist, Hillingdon Hospital, London, UK, M.B.B.S. (Bom), DMRE (BOM), DMRE(Liverpool), FRCR (UK), for his unique chapter on 'Role of Radiology and Imaging in Orthopedics', which is written up to give students an idea of the importance of Radiology and Imaging in Orthopedics. I would thank Dr. Geethan I, M.S. Orth., DNB (Orth), Orthopedic Surgeon, Fellow, Ortho One, Speciality Hospital, Coimbatore, India, and Dr. David V. Rajan, M.S. Orth., MNAMS, FRCS (G) Consultant Orthopedic Surgeon, Director, Ortho One, Coimbatore, India, and Past

President of the Indian Arthroscopy Society for their timely help on the chapter on 'Arthroscopy of the Knee Joint', which was specially written up for this book.

I would like to thank Sharad Goyal, D.Orth. (Gold Med), M.S. Orth., DNB Orth, M.Ch. Orth. (Liv), Orthopedic Surgeon, Department of Trauma & Orthopedics, St Richard's Hospital, Chichester PO19 6SE, West Sussex, UK for his active interest and help in completing my book.

Finally, I would like to thank Dr. Robert H. Cofield, M.D., Emeritus Chairman, Department of Orthopedic Surgery, Mayo Clinic, Professor of Orthopedics, Mayo Clinic College of Medicine, Rochester, MN, for his ever encouraging foreword for this book of mine.

I would like to express my sincere thanks to Springer-Verlag for their kind permission to allow me to reproduce 35 snaps of my book entitled *Clinical Examination in Orthopedics* (Springer) for this book of mine.

Above all I would like to thank Mr. Steffan D. Clements, Editor, Clinical Medicine, Springer (London) for his untiring guidance in the preparation of this book.

I would like to express my sincere gratitude and thanks to all the Orthopedic Surgeons for their valuable contribution in their subspecialities. This textbook is mainly valuable and a must for the beginner who faces Orthopedics as he encounters in daily life, and, when combined with my book entitled *Clinical Examination in Orthopedics* (Springer), would make him complete in all aspects of Orthopedics, both clinical and theoretical.

I am very grateful to my son who has helped me in the tables, corrections, diagrams, charts and formatting of this book and its presentation.

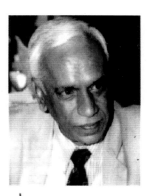

(Dr. K. Mohan Iyer)

Acknowledgements

I am extremely thankful to Dr. Dilip Malhotra, M.S. Orth., M.Ch. Orth., FICS, Consultant Orthopedic Surgeon, International Hospital Bahrain, for his valuable help in clinical photographs and radiographs. I am indebted to Mr. S. Siddiqui, M.S. Orth., FRCSOrth, Consultant Orthopedic Surgeon, Kettering General Hospital, Kettering, UK. for his contribution on the chapter on the Hand and Fingers in Regional Orthopedics and for the chapter on the Hand and Fingers in Orthopedic Trauma. I would like to thank Mr. Shaishav Bhagat M.S. (Ortho), MRCS (Edinburgh), FRCS (Tr. & Orth), Specialist registrar, Kettering General Hospital, UK, who has written the chapters on Polytrauma and Trauma in the Foot and Ankle along with Mr. Bhavik M. Shah M.S. Orth., M.Ch. Orth., FRCSOrth, Consultant Orthopedic Surgeon, Kettering General Hospital, Kettering, UK. I would express my gratitude to Mr. D. K. Menon M.S. Orth. (AIIMS), DNB (Orth), M.Ch. (Orth) Liverpool, FRCS (Tr & Orth).

Honorary Senior Lecturer (Medical Education), University of Leicester

Consultant Orthopedic Surgeon, Kettering General Hospital, Rothwell Road, Kettering, Northamptonshire, NN16 8UZ, England, United Kingdom.

I would also like to thank Mr. Shibu P. Krishnan, Orthopedic Surgeon, M.S. Orth., D.Orth., DNB, MRCS, FRCS (Tr & Orth) for his valuable help in Regional Trauma of Orthopedics involving the Cervical Spine, Thoracolumbar Spine, Sacrum and Coccyx and Scoliosis with Spinal deformities. I am extremely thankful to Dr. Sughran Banerjee, M.B.B.S., AFRCS, Dip. SICOT, Consultant Orthopedic Surgeon for his chapters on Injuries of the thumb in Trauma management in Orthopedics. Above all I am very thankful to Mr. M.A. Syed, Orthopedic Surgeon, Kent, UK. M.B.B.S., MRCSEd, FRCS Orth, for his contribution on "Amputations" in General Orthopedics.

I would like to express my gratitude to Dr. Suhas Namjoshi, MBBS (Bom), DMRE(BOM), DMRE(Liverpool), FRCR (UK) Consultant Radiologist, Hillingdon, UK, for his chapter on Role of Radiology and Imaging in Orthopedics. I am also grateful to Prof. Naresh Shetty, Dean and Professor of Orthopedics, M.S. Ramaiah Medical Teaching Hospital for writing up the chapters on Carpal Tunnel syndrome and Dequervain's stenosing tenovaginitis in Regional Orthopedics and in Fractures of both the bones in the forearm, Monteggia fracture-dislocation, Galeazzi fracture-dislocation, Colles' and Smith's fracture in Trauma in Orthopedics. I am extremely grateful to Magdi E. Greiss, M.D., M.Ch. (Orth), FRCS, Senior Consultant Orthopedic Surgeon North Cumbria University Hospitals UK, Former President, BOFAS (UK) for his valuable collection of X-rays/snaps used in this book. I would like to thank Dr. Sharad Goyal for his chapter on 'The pelvis' in Trauma in Orthopedics, and on the chapter on Total Joint Replacement in General Orthopedics and also thank Mr. Lee J. Taylor, FRCS, Senior Consultant Orthopedic Surgeon, Department of Trauma & Orthopedics, St Richard's Hospital, Chichester PO19 6SE,West Sussex, UK, for his help and encouragement on Total Hip Replacement, and his permission to use the X-rays in this chapter on Total Joint Replacement. I am extremely grateful to Dr. Javad Parvizi, M.D., Rothman Institute, Philadelphia, PA 19107, for permitting us to describe his Parvizi criteria in Infection after Total Joint Replacement and their treatment. I am extremely indebted to Mr. Adhish Avasthi, M.B.B.S., M.S. Orth, MRCS, Registrar Orthopedics and Mr. Richard Hill, M.B. Ch.B., FRCS Ed, FRCS (Tr & Orth) Ed, Consultant Orthopedic Surgeon, Department of Trauma & Orthopedics, St Richard's Hospital, Chichester PO19 6SE,West Sussex, UK, for his comprehensive description on Common Sports Injuries, which is a subspeciality in vogue. I am extremely thankful to Dr Geethan I, M.S. Orth., DNB (Orth), Orthopedic Surgeon and Dr. David V. Rajan M.S. Orth, MNAMS, FRCS(G), Consultant Orthopedic Surgeon, Director, Ortho One, Coimbatore, India, and Past President of the Indian Arthroscopy Society, India for their contribution on the chapter on Arthroscopy of the Knee. Above all, I am extremely grateful to Prof. Naresh Shetty, M.S. Orth, Dean and Professor of Orthopedics, M.S. Ramaiah Medical Teaching Hospital, Bangalore-560 054, India, who along with me has written the chapters on The Wrist Joint in Regional Orthopedics and The Forearm and Wrist in Trauma in Orthopedics.

Contents

Contributors

Adhish Avasthi, MBBS, MS (Orth), MRCS (Glasg)

Sughran Banerjee, AFRCS, Dip. SICOT Apollo Gleneagles Hospital, Kolkata, West Bengal, India

Shaishav Bhagat, M.S. (Ortho), MRCS (Edinburgh), FRCS (Tr. & Orth) Kettering General Hospital, Kettering, UK

I. Geethan, M.S. Orth, DNB(Orth) Ortho One Speciality Hospital, Coimbatore, Tamil Nadu, India

Sharad Goyal, D'Orth (Gold Med), MS'Orth, DNB'Orth, M.Ch.'Orth(Liv) Department of Trauma and Orthopedics, St. Richards Hospital, Chichester, West Sussex, UK

Magdi E. Greiss, MD, MCh (Orth), FRCS North Cumbria University Hospitals, Whitehaven, UK

Former President, BOFAS, UK

Richard Hill, MB ChB, FRCS Ed, FRCS (Tr&Orth) Ed Department of Trauma & Orthopedics, St Richards Hospital, Chichester West Sussex, UK

K. Mohan Iyer Consultant Orthopedic Surgeon, Bangalore University, Bangalore, Karnataka, India

Shibu P. Krishnan, MS.Orth, DNB, D'Orth, MRCS, FRCS (Tr & Orth) London, UK

Dilip Malhotra, MCh. Orth,MS.Orth,FICS International Hospital of Bahrain, Bahrain, Bahrain

Dipen K. Menon, MS Orth (AIIMS), DNB (Orth), MCh (Orth) Liverpool, FRCS (Tr & Orth) Consultant Orthopedic Surgeon, University of Leicester, Leicester, UK

Kettering General Hospital, Kettering, Northamptonshire, UK

Suhas Namjoshi, MBBS (Bom), DMRE (Bom), DMRE (Liverpool) FRCR (UK) Hillingdon (West), London, UK

David V. Rajan, M.S. Orth, MNAMS, FRCS(G) Ortho One, Coimbatore, Tamil Nadu, India

Past President, Indian Arthroscopy Society, Coimbatore, Tamil Nadu, India

Bhavik M. Shah, M.S. Orth, MCh. Orth, FRCS. Orth Kettering General Hospital, Kettering, UK

Naresh Shetty, M.S. Orth M.S. Ramaiah Medical Teaching Hospital, Bangalore, Karnataka, India

Shabih Siddiqui, M.S. Orth, FRCS. Orth Consultant Orthopedic Surgeon, Kettering General Hospital, Kettering, UK

Gyanendra Kumar Singh, MBBS Hons, D.Orth. MSOrth, FRCS Edin, MCh Chichester, UK

M. A. Syed, MBBS, MRCS, Ed., FRCS. Orth Kent, UK

Part I
The Upper Limb

Chapter 1
The Shoulder Joint

K. Mohan Iyer

Acute Synovitis of the Shoulder Joint

Acute synovitis of the shoulder is less common than the knee joint.

It may be caused by injury or due to a local infection such as rheumatism. It may also be found associated in inflammatory conditions of the neighboring tendons and bursae. It may also be seen in the early stages of tuberculosis.

The shoulder joint is swollen and its movements are painful, particularly when the arm is allowed to hang supported only by the muscles and ligaments. This synovial effusion is very well noticed in the delto-pectoral groove, where the joint is usually aspirated. Diagnostic aspiration is usually done between the acromion and the head of the humerus by inserting the needle horizontally and downward and backward.

Sprain of the Shoulder Joint

This happens when the shoulder joint is wrenched beyond the normal limits of its movements. The capsule and the synovial membrane may be torn alone or stretched or in combination. There is usually an extravasation of blood into the peri-articular tissues and it may occasionally involve the tendon sheaths, and these may be followed by peri-articular fibrosis or adhesions.

K.M. Iyer
Consultant Orthopedic Surgeon, Bangalore University,
152, Kailash Apartments 8th Main, Malleswaram 120/H-2K,
560 003 Bangalore, Karnataka, India
e-mail: kmiyer28@hotmail.com

K.M. Iyer (ed.), *Orthopedics of the Upper and Lower Limb*,
DOI 10.1007/978-1-4471-4447-2_1, © Springer-Verlag London 2013

Scapulo-humeral peri-arthritis may be due to:

1. Acute and chronic inflammatory processes, such as bursitis, bicipital tenovaginitis, tendinitis, calcerous deposits, or rheumatic shoulder disease
2. Trauma, contusions, sprains, fractures, dislocations, ruptures of the rotator cuff or the long head of biceps, and tears of the capsule
3. Extensive immobilization for fracture, or infection, or dislocation
4. Referred pain from elsewhere, such as myocardial infarction, cervical spondylosis, or pulmonary lesions

Routinely X-rays are done to exclude any bone damage.

Treatment

Great care should be used to prevent the formation of adhesions. Hence, earliest treatment by physiotherapy along with heat therapy is carried out to ensure the best result. Diathermy and re-education of muscles are carried out in all cases.

Bursitis

Subdeltoid or Subacromial Bursitis

The subacromial bursa lies beneath the upper part of the deltoid muscle and extends below the acromion process. It mainly serves to remove friction and permit rotation of the greater tuberosity of the humerus inward below the acromion process during movements of abduction and rotation of the shoulder.

Inflammation of the bursa nearly always occurs due to a lesion of the neighboring structures, and it is not a structure where the disease starts, but one which limits disease by forming adhesions causing fixation of the parts. Inflammation of the supraspinus tendon may be painless, but when the adjacent bursa is involved, which is richly supplied by nerves and vessels is painful.

Clinical Features

1. Pain at the shoulder on abduction and internal rotation of the humerus, along with severe aching at night, and tenderness at the shoulder.
2. There is usually a tender point over the greater tuberosity of the humerus, which disappears under the acromion on abduction (Dawburn's sign).
3. In some cases, there may be a history of injury to the shoulder, such as a fall on the outstretched arm or on to the shoulder.
4. Radiographs may show calcareous deposits in the supraspinatus tendon.

Subcoracoid Bursitis

The subcoracoid bursa is located between the tip of the coracoid process and the capsule of the shoulder joint, and it may extend up to the lesser tuberosity of the humerus. Clinically the patient may complain of pain in the region of the coracoid along with tenderness over the interval between the two bones. In adhesions, there may be limitation of lateral rotation and abduction. In such cases, a diagnostic injection of 1 % lignocaine and hydrocortisone is very helpful.

The Diagnosis of Shoulder Disabilities

Firstly, a careful detailed accurate history is a must in all shoulder conditions. A radiographic examination is mandatory of both shoulders in a position of lateral rotation, to exclude lesions such as myositis ossificans, loose bodies, and small fractures of the articular surfaces. In addition, an X-ray of the cervical spine is also taken.

Treatment of Shoulder Conditions

While the treatment will vary according to the individual condition, most of them will benefit from the shoulder being rested in the optimal functional position of 75° of abduction along with a small amount of lateral rotation.

Subcoracoid Bursitis: Heat will diminish the inflammation and thereafter postural exercises are very helpful. In very refractory cases, it may be necessary to excise the bursa.

Subacromial Bursitis: Mild cases may be helped by an injection of lignocaine and hydrocortisone into the bursa along with the arm rested in an a splint.

In refractory cases, the bursa may be excised along with removal of the calcareous depositis.

Lesions of the Supraspinatus Tendon

The superior and posterior portions of the capsule of the shoulder joint are strengthened by the incorporation of flat expanded tendons of the supraspinatus, the infraspinatus, and the teres minor tendon. All together form the rotator cuff and this is separated from the deltoid and the acromion process by the subdeltoid bursa.

The supraspinatus tendon lies superiorly forming the roof of the joint and the floor of the subacromial bursa.

Complete rupture of its tendon usually occurs close to the greater tuberosity, which leaves a direct communication gap between the bursa and the joint, which varies between 1 and 6 cm.

In addition to this, smaller tears may occur involving only a few fibers.

Etiology

Along with every abduction movement, there is some friction and contact between supraspinatus tendon and the acromion. The subdeltoid bursa because of its location minimizes the friction. With advancing age, there is degeneration of the supraspinatus tendon, due to repeated minor trauma, when the fibers become worn away and a tendinitis occurs. Since the tendon is vascular, calcareous deposits may occur resulting in calcification leading to a partial or complete rupture of the tendon.

Tendinitis of the Supraspinatus Tendon

The symptom complex often follows a history of minor injury, with the patient presenting with pain over the shoulder at the deltoid insertion. Movements are not usually limited in the initial stages. However, the arc of abduction between 60° and 120° is very painful and is the apparent point where the tender area impinges on the acromion. Radiographs show no abnormality. In arthritis, pain remains continuously throughout the movement, as well as rotations.

Treatment

In the early stages, physiotherapy and heat with pendulum exercises are helpful. For night pain, the arm is immobilized in a sling or a circular body bandage.

Good results are obtained by the injection of lignocaine with hydrocortisone and hyaluronidase into the tender area.

Calcification of the Supraspinatus Tendon

The occurrence of calcareous deposits over lying the greater tuberosity of the humerus is seen in some cases and may give pain when they extend to beneath the bursal wall, which is richly supplied with nerves and blood vessels. It may also cause no symptoms when it lies deep in tendinous structure.

The condition may occur at all ages usually with a history of injury. There may be acute pain with gradually increasing stiffness.

The X-ray appearances are characteristic. There is a small discrete uneven and irregular shadow over the greater tuberosity in the region of the supraspinatus tendon (Fig. 1.1). It can be differentiated from a loose body as it is far too intra-articular. In addition, the greater tuberosity may show some degree of osteoporosis.

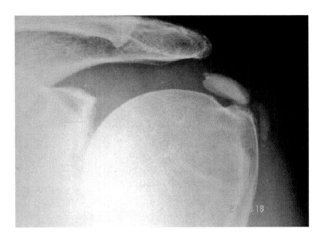

Fig. 1.1 Anteroposterior radiograph of the shoulder showing supraspinatus calcification (Courtesy: Dilip Malhotra, Bahrain) (Reproduced with kind permission of Springer Verlag)

Pathology

The material consists of a non-crystalline, calcareous matter embedded in a mass of inflammatory cells containing foreign body giant cells. Cultures taken during operation are sterile and biochemical examination shows amorphous calcium carbonate and phosphate. The material in the early stages is like a tooth paste and later on becomes calcareous.

Treatment

In acute cases, immobilization in an abduction splint or a sling is enough to prevent dependency of the limb, which is associated with disappearance of the deposit and subsidence of inflammation. At the same time, short wave diathermy or radiant heat with active exercises are helpful.

Considerable success may be obtained by aspiration and irrigation of the lesion with normal saline.

The results of surgical excision of the deposits are reliable and definite.

The mass may be too thick to be evacuated by aspiration, though it can be tried first.

In refractory and chronic cases, a total acromionectomy may be helpful.

Incomplete Rupture of the Supraspinatus Tendon

This occurs in 30 % of the patients and it is usually a common sequel to tendinitis.

Pain is over the shoulder and tenderness is also present over the tendon.

Immobilization in an abduction splint is very useful in the early stages.

In cases where there is no improvement, the tendon is exposed by an operation and the tear is dealt like a complete rupture.

When there is evidence of a tear, the subdeltoid bursa is fully explored and the bursal wall removed.

Rupture of the Supraspinatus Tendon and the Rotator Cuff

The actual tear may be painless, and it is diagnosed by immediate weakness of the arm, with the patient unable to abduct the shoulder. Local tenderness may be elicited over the greater tuberosity, which disappears under the acromion. Coarse crepitation may be heard in the region of the bursa and by a characteristic abduction syndrome.

Diagnosis

The diagnostic sign is a greater limitation of active than of passive abduction, in the presence of a functioning deltoid. Abduction cannot be carried out by the deltoid alone, and the supraspinatus is an essential synergist.

An arthrography by injecting a radio-opaque dye will help in outlining the severity of the rupture.

Certain signs and symptoms indicate a complete rupture of the supraspinatus and these should be present within 24 h of injury as follows:

1. Occupation – labor
2. Age – over 40 years
3. No symptoms in the shoulder prior to the accident
4. Adequate injury – usually a fall
5. Immediate sharp and brief pain
6. Severe pain on following night
7. Loss of power in elevation of the arm
8. Negative X-ray
9. Little, if any, restriction when stooping
10. Faulty scapulo-humeral rhythm
11. A tender spot
12. A sulcus
13. An eminence
14. At the insertion of the suprapinatus
15. Which causes a jog
16. A wince
17. Soft crepitus as the tuberosity
18. Disappears under the acromion when the arm is elevated, and usually reappears during descent of the arm

Treatment

It should be emphasized that an immediate suture is a simple and successful operation. Delay means retraction of the tendon along with a much more serious problem.

The ruptured tendon should be repaired by an operation, after freshening the gaps and sutured with strong chromic catgut or silk.

Post-operatively the arm is immobilized in a splint with the arm abducted to 90° and laterally rotated to 60° for 4–6 weeks.

Frozen Shoulder or Adhesive Capsulitis

This condition accounts for most of the cases of shoulder disability, in a proportion of 3–2. It affects males usually at a slightly older age group than tendinitis.

The patient gives a history of a painful catch in the region of the shoulder and arm for several months. Gradually he becomes aware of his inability to perform certain tasks, because of stiffness of the arm. Night pain keeping him awake is a frequent complaint. Stiffness in the shoulder gradually increases until all movements are lost.

On examination, there is marked restriction of mainly abduction and rotations and radiographs are normal.

Treatment

Active exercises are advocated in the early stages and no manipulation or forceful passive exercises is advised. Radiant heat and short-wave diathermy is very helpful. Injection of lignocaine with hydrocortisone is helpful in certain cases. Analgesia with anti-inflammatory drugs, such as phenylbutazone or indomethacin, improves the range of movements in some cases.

Recurrent Dislocation of the Shoulder Joint

This condition is common in athletes and epileptics, usually between the ages of 20 and 30 years. The patient is considerably handicapped as the limb loses its power and efficiency.

Fig. 1.2 Anteroposterior
radiograph showing an
anterior dislocation of the
right shoulder (Courtesy:
Dilip Malhotra, Bahrain)
(Reproduced with kind
permission of Springer
Verlag)

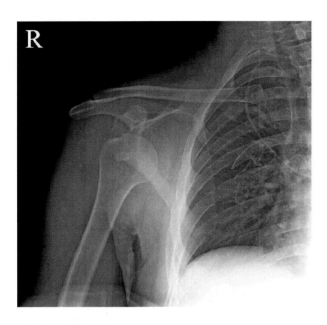

Anterior Dislocations of the Shoulder

There are mainly two types of anterior dislocations of the shoulder, namely:

1. Traumatic type, which constitutes nearly 95 % of all cases, when there is a definite history of injury and the instability is only in one direction.
2. Non-traumatic, which forms the remaining 5 % of the cases, where there is no history of injury, and poor muscular development along with anatomical variations is the main cause, and the results of surgery are unpredictable.

Pathology

In majority of the cases, the initial injury results in detachment of the glenoid labrum and capsule from the anterior aspect of the glenoid, and the displaced head strips the periosteum from the neck of the scapula (Fig. 1.2). Thereafter with recurrent displacement of the humeral head, a defect is produced in the posterolateral aspect of the humeral head. This is of the nature of an impaction fracture produced on the head where it is meets the anterior margin of the glenoid. This is seen on radiographs as a groove or a depression at the upper and outer margin of the humeral head, which is visible with the X-rays taken in internal rotation of 50°. This is often known as the Hill-Sack's lesion.

The detachment of the glenoid capsule and periosteum occurs in nearly 80 % of all cases.

The initial reduction is reduced and the arm held immobilized in full internal rotation and adduction for a period of 4 weeks.

Symptoms

The dislocation finally becomes painless. Considerable muscular atrophy may be seen in the muscles around the shoulder, particularly the brachialis, triceps, deltoid, the supra- and the infraspinatus.

Treatment

Operative treatment is mainly advisable when the dislocation recurs more than three times.

Bankart Operation

Since the basic pathology is a detachment of the anterior glenoid labrum, this procedure is mainly meant to repair this defect.

The shoulder joint is opened by a delto-pectoral incision with an osteotomy of the coracoid process. Lateral rotation of the humerus exposes the subscapularis and this muscle is divided about 2 cm from its insertion .The anterior detached margin of the glenoid is then identified and freshened to be relocated at its original place by silk sutures. The subscapularis and the wound is closed and post-operatively the arm is immobilized for 6 weeks, before gentle exercises are begun with intensive physiotherapy thereafter.

The main difficulty is to drill holes in the glenoid for suture with silk, because the glenoid is at a considerable depth in the wound.

Capsulorrhappy

This operation is conventionally called as the Putti Platt procedure after their description initially. The shoulder joint is opened as usual and the subscapularis muscle identified. The muscles are then divided near its insertion and then double breasted with the arm held in internal rotation, for 6 weeks, after which physiotherapy is started.

Both the above operations carry a recurrence rate of 5–8 %. Considerable variations have been used for stabilizing the anterior aspect of the shoulder during surgery.

Posterior Dislocation of the Shoulder

Even in the traumatic cases, this dislocation is very rare. In this condition, the shoulder is locked in adduction and internal rotation, with the humeral head being palpable posteriorly.

Radiographs show the absence of the usual half moon shadow of the humeral head overlapping the glenoid fossa and this is confirmed by the axillary view.

In this condition, the glenoid labrum is detached posteriorly and the grooved defect is located anteriorly on the humeral head.

Treatment is by closed reduction and immobilization in some adduction and maximum external rotation for 3 weeks followed by physiotherapy.

The operation of repairing the coraco-clavicular ligament using non-absorbable sutures and temporary transfixation of the joint by a thick Kirschner wire for 4–6 weeks gives encouraging results.

Surgical reconstruction with a metallic prosthesis is usually rarely out because of a difficulty in restoring abduction power, due to interference with the insertion of the rotator cuff into the greater tuberosity.

Snapping Shoulder

This condition produces an audible click in certain movements of the shoulder, and it may result from a voluntary subluxation of the shoulder joint or by a tendon slipping over a bony prominence, for example, the short tendon of the biceps over the lesser tuberosity.

This condition may later on become habitual or involuntary, and sometimes the patient can produce the sound on request.

Snapping Scapula

This is a condition of grating or snapping of the scapula, due to some anomalous condition between the ribs and the under surface of the scapula. There may be a loud snap or a fine grating sound which may be divided into three main groups:

1. Those due to changes in the bony structure of the under surface of the scapula or of the wall of the chest
2. Those with changes in the musculature between the scapula and the chest wall
3. Those with changes in the bursae normally present or abnormally present between the scapula and the chest wall

Bone Causes

1. The tubercle of luschka: It is a small bony prominence located in the anterior aspect of the superior angle of the scapula, and it is usually the size of a pea, usually covered by a bursa.
2. Abnormal curvature of the superior angle of the scapula, which is congenital in origin.
3. Scapular snapping has been noted in exostoses of the ribs or on the under surface of the scapula. The exostoses may be found on the superior angle or inferior angle of the scapula and may vary in size from a nodule to a mushroom-shaped mass.
4. Tumors of the ribs or scapula, fracture of the either, angulation or buckling of the ribs.

Muscular Causes

The second main group is that associated with changes in the muscles lying between the scapula and the ribs.

Bursal Causes

The third main group is that scapular snapping has been attributed to the presence of normal or adventitious bursae. Normally two are present beneath the scapula, one at the upper angle, situated in the depth of the serratus anterior muscle and this is present in one in eight persons. The other, which is somewhat rare, is found in the connective tissue between the serratus anterior and the upper part of the lateral wall of the chest.

Winged Scapula

This is a deformity which is fairly well recognized as secondary in some cases of paralysis of the serratus anterior. Though some people believe that it is caused by a rupture of the muscle at the scapular insertion.

The long thoracic nerve arises from the 5th, 6th, and 7th cervical nerves, with the upper two piercing the scaleus medius and the 7th nerve passing in front of the muscle. The three nerve roots unite at the level of the first rib to form one single trunk which descends along the inner wall of the axilla, behind the brachial plexus and the axillary vessels and upon the lateral aspect of the serratus, to which it is distributed.

The function of the serratus anterior is mainly to fix the scapula to the thorax when the arm is elevated, particularly anteriorly and also to rotate the scapula in abduction and during forward elevation of the arm at the shoulder.

Hence, the nerve is liable to be damaged at:

1. The suprascapular region from sudden or protracted trauma, e.g., carrying heavy weights on the shoulder
2. In the axilla from direct force
3. At the level of the union of its three roots, due to abnormalities of the first rib
4. From violent contraction of the scalenus medius muscle, such as in swimming, a vigorous swing at the punching bag which misses, a violent pull up when starting a car
5. Possibly in the axilla due to pressure from enlarged glands

Also there exists a group of cases following typhoid, measles, influenza, and an injection of anti-tetanic serum.

The earliest symptom is pain along the base of the neck and downward over the scapula and deltoid. A common symptom is the patient's fatigue on elevating the arm or inability to do this fully. This weakness may pass unnoticed by the patient himself, and abnormal prominence of the vertebral border of the scapula is a sign more frequently observed by others than the patient himself.

On examination of the patient, the main clinical observation is that there is weakness of the pushing power of the affected shoulder, along with weakness of the abducting power of the arm above the horizontal plane.

Winging of the scapula is always present when the arm is fully abducted or elevated anteriorly.

Tenderness may be present over the course of the long thoracic nerve, the maximal point being the mid-axillary line in the fourth intercostal space.

The affected scapula is near the midline and may overlap the vertebral column when the arm is abducted.

Treatment

It may be conservation or operative.

Numerous types of conservative measures have been tried, such as the arm is immobilized in a plaster shoulder spica case in order to relax the muscles followed by physiotherapy. The best position for the arm to be fixed is abduction and lateral rotation, with backward displacement of the shoulder girdle, so holding the scapula close to the thoracic wall.

Operative Treatment

Some means of anchoring the scapula seem to be the ideal way to relieve the symptoms. Various methods have been devised for this, such as four strips of fascia are used to sling the scapula to holes drilled in the spinous processes from the fourth to the seventh dorsal vertebra.

An alternative procedure is transplanting the teres major muscle to the digitations of the serratus, while a similar result can be obtained by using a portion of the pectoralis major muscle. A further alternative procedure is transferring the teres major into the sixth and seventh ribs anteriorly with restoration of function.

Neuralgic Amyotrophy (The Shoulder-Girdle Syndrome)

This is a condition characterized by pain and flaccid paralysis of the muscles around the shoulder girdle, which is now very rare and was common in 1939–1945.

Recovery of 70–80 % of normal power occurs.

Etiology

A virus has been suggested, but the absence of constitutional symptoms does not support this theory.

A similar condition occurs after injection of a serum injection, and it is probable that a condition allied to urticaria resulting in perineural edema of the affected roots and nerves comparable to the urticaria of serum sickness.

Symptoms

The onset is not usually accompanied by constitutional symptoms, while pain is normally the presenting symptom. The pain is localized to the back of the scapula and may go up or down the neck. This pain lasts for about 14 days, when it suddenly stops and muscular paralysis then sets in.

A striking feature is the rapid development of muscular weakness after a variable period of pain. The weakness is of a lower motor neurone type with flaccidity of the affected muscles often with rapid wasting. Fasciculation is never seen. The pathological process is in one or more peripheral nerves, while in others it may be in the nerve root, and in some cases there may be a lesion in the spinal cord.

The nerves frequently affected are the long thoracic and suprascapular and circumflex nerves. The common nerve roots to be affected are the 5th and 6th cervical with weakness of the spinati, deltoid, biceps, supinator longus and at times the clavicular head of the pectoralis major. There is impairment of the biceps and supinator jerks along with sensory impairment over a strip on the outer side of the arm and forearm.

In certain cases, there is patchy muscle wasting and weakness which is not corresponding to any nerve or nerve roots, and in these cases, a spinal cord involvement is suspected. Sensory changes may occur in many cases. The CSF and radiographs are normal.

Differential Diagnosis

1. Anterior poliomyelitis must be excluded by the fact that the CSF is normal and there are no constitutional upsets, while sensory changes are present.
2. Prolapsed disc usually affects one root. The profound weakness and atrophy of the shoulder-girdle syndrome does not occur.
3. Localized paralysis and wasting of muscles are not features of brachial neuritis.
4. Progressive muscular atrophy may be excluded, because of the features of acute onset with pain, the rapid development of wasting, the absence of fasciculation, and the non-progressive course of the disease, as well as by the sensory changes that are often present.

Treatment

No specific treatment for the condition is known, and it may be treated like poliomyelitis with analgesics and splints to rest the muscles. It is very important to put the shoulder joint through the full range of movements at least twice a day to prevent stiffness.

Dropped Shoulder

In this condition, there is injury to the spinal accessory nerve resulting in paralysis of the trapezius muscle as is seen in direct trauma, traction lesions, or its use as a nerve pedicle transfer for facial paralysis or after an operation on the posterior triangle or during radical neck dissection for cancer.

Here the patients complain of a dragging sensation about the shoulder girdle including loss of shoulder abduction beyond 90°. On examination, the affected shoulder will have dropped with the clavicle taking up a more horizontal position. The scapula is displaced laterally and inferiorly as well as being rotated outward away from the midline.

Conservative measures are adopted at an early stage, but if not responding then an operation can be considered by using a strip of fascia lata sling of the medial region to the spinous processes of thoracic 1 and 2 vertebrae and the outward transfer of the levator scapulae muscle to the lateral part of the scapular spine.

Spontaneous Axillary Vein Thrombosis

This condition may appear in a normal young human being when the upper arm becomes diffusely swollen and discolored. Eighty percent of the cases are males, and 70 % have the right arm affected.

The condition is often due to trauma, such as a man vigorously scrubbing his back in a bath, or when the patient has strained his arm jumping from a tractor. The initial injury is usually accompanied by acute pain and thereafter the arm becomes limp and useless. The whole limb swells up rapidly and there is difficulty in moving the shoulder and to a lesser degree the elbow. Superficial veins of the arm become distended and obvious along with a tingling sensation in the fingers. Firstly, the pain is of the stabbing type which changes to a dull intermittent type later on. The hand and arm usually assume a dusky hue.

On examination, the veins of the arm, hand, and pectoral region are prominent and engorged in appearance, particularly at the acromio-thoracic anastomosis. There is marked tenderness of the axillary veins and the radiographs are normal. There are no motor or sensory changes seen.

Venography is carried out into the median cubital vein which shows the site of obstruction.

Treatment

The patient is treated in bed with the arm elevated and exercises within the limits of comfort. Anti-coagulation therapy is started with heparin at once and controlled and monitored by the clotting time.

Some people have suggested an anatomic abnormality where the phrenic nerve passes in front of the subclavian vein, giving rise to compression by pressure against the scalenus anterior tendon, just like a ligature. Recovery mainly depends on collateral circulation and this depends on whether the nerve passes medial or lateral to the external jugular vein and the thrombus formation. It may be that after the anti-coagulant treatment, a simple operation of section of the phrenic nerve may be helpful.

Chapter 2
The Arm

K. Mohan Iyer

Muscular Strains in the Shoulder Region

The muscles in the shoulder region which are commonly injured are the deltoid, the biceps, the medial rotators, and very rarely the lateral rotators.

Muscular lesions are recognizable by the fact that (1) the muscle is painful when actively moved, (2) when resistance is offered to it during movement, and (3) when the muscle is passively stretched.

The Deltoid

Gross rupture of the muscle is unusual, but rupture of a group of fibers is usually seen.

When the muscle is strained, active abduction is very painful and diminished, though passive abduction can be carried out.

When the patient is asked to hold the abducted arm in position, acute pain is felt and the arm falls to one side.

The Supraspinatus

Injury to this muscle is very important.

K.M. Iyer
Consultant Orthopedic Surgeon, Bangalore University,
152, Kailash Apartments 8th Main, Malleswaram 120/H-2K,
560 003 Bangalore, Karnataka, India
e-mail: kmiyer28@hotmail.com

K.M. Iyer (ed.), *Orthopedics of the Upper and Lower Limb*,
DOI 10.1007/978-1-4471-4447-2_2, © Springer-Verlag London 2013

The Biceps

The main function of the biceps is to supinate the forearm, and flex the arm at the shoulder joint, and flexion at the elbow joint is a secondary effect.

Bicepital lesions rarely take the form of complete division of the muscle bellies and there is swelling or a swelling when the muscle contracts.

Rupture of the Long Head of Biceps

This is a rare, but very occasional lesion.

In most cases, there is a history of injury, which may be in the form of lifting heavy weights or violent extension of the forearm while flexion is being carried out, while in a few cases, it may also be spontaneous.

The clinical features are characteristic, when the muscle belly shows a bulbous enlargement in its lateral half, when compared to the opposite side.

Treatment

Treatment is usually by operation and the results are satisfactory.

The rupture is exposed through an anterolateral incision and the cut ends identified, with the cut ends being sutured end to end with the elbow held flexed.

Tears of the rotator cuff can be identified by extending the incision proximally, and this is repaired by an end to end suture.

At times, there is an avulsion of the distal end of the biceps from the coracoid process, and when length permits is fixed to the bony insertion.

Recurrent dislocation of the long head of biceps may occur following a tear of the bicipital fascia.

The Medial Rotators

The muscles responsible for this movement is the pectoralis major and the subscapularis.

In strains of these muscles, pain is experienced on active medial rotation, and the movement is usually restricted.

The Lateral Rotators

Injury or strains of these muscles is very rare and may usually result from traction on the muscles. Lateral rotation is usually done by the teres minor and the infraspinatus.

Bicipital Tendinitis

The long tendon of the biceps is very intimate with the articular capsule of the shoulder joint and hence is readily affected in inflammatory processes affecting the shoulder joint. It also has a synovial sheath contained within the transverse ligament and this in turn can undergo an inflammatory change.

The main symptoms are pain in the shoulder joint which is located over the bicipital groove and can be aggravated by forced resistance to flexion of the elbow joint and supination of the forearm.

The pathologic process may go on till the tendon becomes atrophic and ruptures.

Conservative treatment is in the form of short wave diathermy, injection of hydrocortisone and rest to the arm.

It had a much better prognosis than chronic inflammations involving the shoulder joint itself.

Dislocation of the Biceps Brachii

This condition has been recognized for a long time. The tendon is usually anchored in place by the attachment of the articular capsule just proximal to the lesser tuberosity, and the medial ridge of the bicipital sulcus which is often very deep. This condition may result by a violent muscular action that may dislocate the tendon, which results in the tendon slipping over the lesser tuberosity decreasing the tension of the muscle giving rise to the classical bicipital syndrome.

The symptoms are usually acute resembling a ruptured biceps tendon, with the pain in the region of the bicipital groove, which is increased on external rotation, when the muscle belly is flabby and lower than in the normal position.

The diagnosis is not always easy, as the patient can produce this condition by bringing the extended arm to overhead extension and lateral rotation holding a 5-lb weight in each hand, when the examiner puts a finger on the tendon and may feel or hear the snap.

Chapter 3
The Elbow

K. Mohan Iyer

Tennis Elbow

This troublesome condition is considered by some people to be a form of radio-humeral bursitis, as the exact nature of the condition is not known. This condition is also known as "epicondylitis" or "epicondylalgia."

The condition occurs in others than tennis players, such as housewives, violin players, etc.

Clinical Features

Rarely does it have a sudden origin and is accompanied by a definite swelling over the origin of the extensor tendons. More frequently does it appear after prolonged and constant exercises, which has necessitated continuous flexion and extension of the elbow and pronation and supination of the forearm.

Tenderness is usually present on the lateral or anterior aspect of the lateral condyle of the humerus. The pain is very persistent and becomes a nuisance in some patients. There is also a sense of weakness when attempts are made to do any lifting movements.

Examination shows little more than an area of definite tenderness. In most cases, the elbow cannot be fully extended and any attempt made to force this is also painful. On active movement with the wrist palmar flexed, there is pain at the site of the lesion, particularly when the forearm is pronated and the elbow flexed. Radiographs of the elbow are normal.

K.M. Iyer
Consultant Orthopedic Surgeon, Bangalore University,
152, Kailash Apartments 8th Main, Malleswaram 120/H-2K,
560 003 Bangalore, Karnataka, India
e-mail: kmiyer28@hotmail.com

K.M. Iyer (ed.), *Orthopedics of the Upper and Lower Limb,*
DOI 10.1007/978-1-4471-4447-2_3, © Springer-Verlag London 2013

There are many theories to the pathology of this condition as:

1. Traumatic periostitis
2. Tear of the origin of the common extensor tendons with supervening fibrosis
3. Actual bursitis
4. Hypertrophy of the synovial fringes
5. Part played by the orbicular ligament in the production of pain, since resection of the ligament gives relief in some cases
6. Some also believe that contracture of the extensor carpi radialis brevis may be the cause of pain as Z-plasty lengthening of this tendon above the level of the synovial sheath in the forearm gives relief in some cases

Treatment

In acute cases, rest from the causative factor gives immediate relief and cure in some cases. A cock-up splint given to the wrist joint also helps in some cases, by decreasing the tension on extensor tendon.
Some form of physical treatment like short wave diathermy and heat may be helpful in some cases.

In some cases, manipulation of the elbow in complete extension by the forearm fully pronated and the wrist and fingers flexed may give relief in many cases with an audible click.

Good results may be obtained in some cases by the injection of a local anesthetic and hyaluronidase along with hydrocortisone.

In extremely refractory cases, an operation may be carried out which consists of cutting down to bone along with raising the common extensor origin along with the periosteum. In very occasional cases, an adventitious bursa or a hypertrophied fringe when found may be removed.

Cubitus Varus

This condition is also called as "Gun-stock deformity." It is most commonly seen in a supracondylar fracture. The deformity looks rather ugly with the hand brushing the body in walking (Fig. 3.1).

The deformity can be treated by an operation of wedge osteotomy of the distal humerus. Post-operatively, the arm is treated in a plaster cast with the elbow held in full extension and slight valgus.

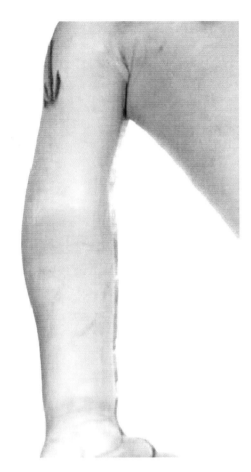

Fig. 3.1 Clinical photograph of cubitus varus (Courtesy: Dilip Malhotra, Bahrain) (Reproduced with kind permission of Springer Verlag)

Cubitus Valgus

This condition is commonly seen in non-union of the fractured lateral condyle. It is seen as a lump on the lateral side of the joint and is a frequent cause of tardy ulnar palsy.

This is mainly noticed by the patient as weakness of the hand along with numbness and tingling of the fingers.

The deformity per se does not require treatment, and if very disabling may be treated operatively by anterior transposition of the ulnar nerve to the front of the elbow.

Tuberculosis of the Elbow

See Chapter 7 in my book entitled 'General principles of Orthopedics and Trauma' (Springer).

Osteoarthritis of the Elbow

See Chapter 5 in my book entitled 'General principles of Orthopedics and Trauma' (Springer).

Ulnar Neuritis of the Elbow

See Chapter 8 in my book entitled 'General principles of Orthopedics and Trauma' (Springer).

Bursitis of the Elbow

See Chapter 17 in my book entitled 'General principles of Orthopedics and Trauma' (Springer)

Sports Elbows

Golfer's Elbow

This condition is commonly seen in golfers, where the common flexor origin over the medial epicondyle are affected just a tennis elbow.

Javelin Thrower's Elbow

This condition is commonly seen in javelin throwers who use an over arm action to throw a javelin, thus resulting in an avulsion injury of the tip of the olecranon. They may also avulse the medial collateral ligament with a round-arm action in throwing a javelin.

Baseball pitchers may suffer extensive elbow damage with hypertrophy of the lower humerus, which no longer fits into the olecranon.

The junior equivalent which is called as a "little leaguer's elbow" is caused by partial avulsion of the medial epicondyle.

Loose Bodies

Its causes may be:

1. *Injury*: A fracture or dislocation, or minor injury when repeated may break off a small piece of bone into the joint resulting in a loose body. Osteochondritis dissecans when detached comes from the capitulum and is probably traumatic in origin.
2. *Degeneration*: In osteoarthritis, small osteophytes may break off, while in Charcot's disease, large pieces of bone may be found in the joint.
3. *Inflammation*: Small fibrinous loose bodies may occur in inflammatory conditions, but the main inflammatory process overshadows the loose bodies.
4. *Idiopathic*: Synovial osteochondromatosis occasionally occurs resulting in multiple loose bodies.

The patient may complain of locking and unlocking of the joint. At times, symptoms of osteoarthritis may co-exist. A loose body is rarely palpable, but when degenerative changes are present, diminution of movements may be found. Radiographs may show the loose body. If they are troublesome, they may be removed. Only in special cases of osteochondritis dissecans there may be a rarefied cystic area in the capitulum along with enlargement of the radial head.

Flail Elbow

There are three main causes of this condition:

1. *Gunshot wound*: There is a scar and often an ulnar nerve palsy. Radiographs show the lesion.
2. *Charcot's disease*: In this condition, there is frailness, but there is no scar and no ulnar nerve palsy.
3. *Poliomyelitis*: With a balanced paralysis the elbow may be flail, it is not the presenting symptom.

Post-traumatic Stiffness

Temporary stiffness may follow any elbow injury. Permanent stiffness may result in limitation of movements, such as severe fractures in young adults or when an injury is complicated by myositis ossificans. Unless the fracture is recent, there is no warmth and tenderness. Radiographs may reveal the old fracture along with myositis ossificans.

Treatment is by rest to achieve a cold elbow and passive movements are prohibited. If myositis ossification is suspected, the elbow is approached bilaterally and the myositic mass removed. The elbow is then transfixed by a metallic pin or a thick K wire with the elbow held in 90 degrees of flexion, which is removed after 3 weeks and active mobilization started. Usually this procedure gives useful movements in the functional arc of the elbow, necessary for day to day function.

Chapter 4
The Forearm

K. Mohan Iyer

Congenital Absence of the Radius

There are varying degrees of hypoplasia or deformity with or without synostosis.

Pathology

Usually the entire radius is absent, but sometimes the defect is only partial when a small portion of the radius remains, generally the upper end. When a small fragment of the radius remains, the ulna may be fused to it, giving rise to a form of radio-ulnar synostosis. This ulna may attain a considerable size in many cases, and is short, thick, and curved, with the concavity of the curvature always toward the radial side of the forearm.

The carpal bones may also show associated abnormalities and usually the scaphoid is absent or a fusion of the scaphoid with neighboring carpal bones. More rarely the lunate is absent.

When the radius is absent, the biceps are usually inserted into the lacertus fibrosus, though in some cases the muscle may be completely absent or fused with the brachialis or coracobrachialis . The brachialis is absent in 50 % of the cases, and when present is usually short and stout and appears to be a continuation of the short head of biceps. Occasionally, it may be continuous with the extensor carpi radialis longus and the two may be inserted into the ulna. The extensor carpi radialis longus and brevis are frequently absent or may be fused with the extensor digitorum communis, while the extensor pollicis may be absent or fused with the neighboring tissues. The

K.M. Iyer
Consultant Orthopedic Surgeon, Bangalore University,
152, Kailash Apartments 8th Main, Malleswaram 120/H-2K,
560 003 Bangalore, Karnataka, India
e-mail: kmiyer28@hotmail.com

K.M. Iyer (ed.), *Orthopedics of the Upper and Lower Limb*,
DOI 10.1007/978-1-4471-4447-2_4, © Springer-Verlag London 2013

flexor pollicis longus and the pronator quadratus are rarely present. The radial nerve usually terminates at the elbow and there is often no radial artery.

Clinical Features

Generally the affected arm shows some degree of atrophy but is most marked in the forearm, which is invariably short, stubby, and bowed with a posterior convexity, and the hand is small and atrophic. Further, it may be deviated to the radial side and slightly palmar flexed, when it is called as a radio-palmar club-hand. The thumb is occasionally absent, and despite these deformities the limb may retain a surprisingly good function, though the grasping power is usually impaired.

Treatment

Usually there is a cosmetic deformity which can be improved upon. Grasp is often accomplished by using the hand against the upper arm. Whatever growth has been obtained is negated by the curvature of the ulna.

The main aim should be to overcome the radial deviation and proximal progression of the carpus as soon as the deformity is recognized. This is accomplished by progressive casting to push the hand over the distal ulnar styloid, which normally takes about 6 weeks. At this point, it can be brought in line or slightly beyond the ulna, but when not held in this position may have a tendency to pop back into the former position. This can be avoided by a holding splint which is molded along the ulna with Velcro straps pulling the hand into the corrected position.

The best results are obtained permanently when carried out below the age of 1. A pin fixation with external support may be given post-operative for 6 weeks, followed by the continued external support for approximately 1 year, or until there is no recurrence of the deformity. If bowing of the ulna fails to straighten with growth, it can always be osteotomized at a later date.

Congenital Absence of the Ulna

This condition is also called as post-axial ulnar hemimelia. It is more common and uncommon than absence of the radius and is more difficult to treat also. Usually there is a union with the radius with the humerus along with marked bowing of the radius. This is usually treated by resection of the cartilaginous analog of the ulna and removed and an arthroplasty attempted through the lower end of the humerus with a sheet of soft tissue.

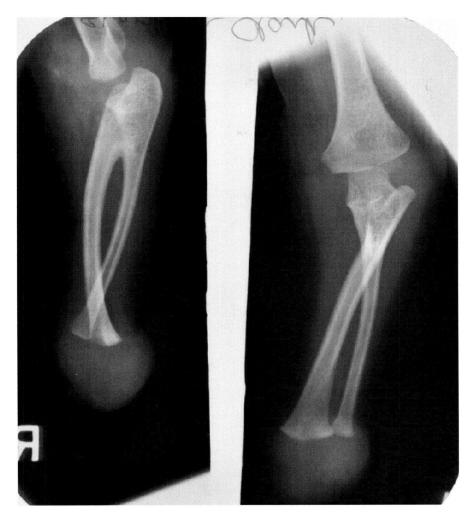

Fig. 4.1 Congenital radio-ulnar synostosis (Courtesy: Magdi E. Greiss, Whitehaven, Cumbria, UK)

Congenital Radio-Ulnar Synostosis

In this condition, one or both the forearms may be fixed at birth in a position mid-way between supination and pronation, usually by fusion of the proximal ends of the radius and ulna. It is equal in both sexes and may have a hereditary tendency.

There are three types of synostosis that can occur:

1. *The true congenital radio-ulnar synostosis*: Here the upper end of the radius is imperfectly formed and fused to the ulna for a varying distance and appears to grow from the upper end. The shaft of the radius arches forward (Fig. 4.1) more

than usual and is longer and stouter than the ulna, suggesting that there has been some arrest in the growth of the ulna or stimulation in the growth of the radius. In over 80 % of the cases, it is bilateral.

2. Here there is a congenital dislocation of the ill-formed radius, and the radius and ulna are anchored at some point short to both the extremities between both the bones, at the coronoid process by a short thick interosseous ligament. The radius is relatively longer and stouter than the ulna, but shows the same curvature as in the primary type. This form is not a true synostosis, but still it does show a trace of movement.

3. In this condition, the head of the radius is present but malformed and together with the upper part of the shaft is fused with the upper end of the ulna.

Etiology

Congenital radio-ulnar synostosis is essentially an arrest of development. The radius and the ulna develop from a single mass of mesoderm as two separate cartilaginous rods. From the 5th week the volar aspect of the developing arm is applied to the trunk, so that the radial and ulnar cartilaginous rods are in a position midway to supination and pronation. If normal separation into distinct rods does not occur at the upper end of the developing bones or if chondrification and later on ossification extends across the mesoderm-filled interval between their upper ends, then a congenital radio-ulnar synostosis develops.

Clinical Features

The classical picture is that the forearm is fixed in a mid-prone position, though the movements of the elbow are free and extension is limited. Wrist movements are usually free. There is no movement between the radius and the ulna.

In the unilateral case, the affected forearm is thinner and has a curious twisted appearance, due to an alteration in the axis of the principal groups of muscles. At the point normally occupied by the head of the radius, there may be a well-defined sulcus, owing to the head being backward or forward and the limitation in the forearm movement is to some extent compensated by rotation of the humerus, but the palm cannot be fully supinated. There is normally no complaint since the normal use of the hand has never been experienced.

Treatment

Though it seems obvious that an operation is indicated, the bony deformity is only a part of the deformity and the soft tissues are not normally developed and the results of operation are indeed disappointing. In the type associated with dislocation of the head of the radius, where the soft parts are normal, the prospect is more hopeful. If the pronation is extreme, it can be reduced by an osteotomy.

Congenital Subluxation of the Wrists (Madelung's Deformity)

Inferior radio-ulnar dislocations of which Madelung's deformity is a type are classified as follows:

1. With fracture
2. Without fracture

    – *Congenital*: Madelung's deformity
    – *Acquired*: Traumatic or Pathological

In this deformity there is defective development of the inner third of the growth cartilage at the distal end of the radius. This results in stunted growth of the epiphysis and diaphysis on the inner side, while growth on the outer two-thirds continues and as a result of which the radial shaft is bowed backward, the interosseous space is increased and the distal end of the ulna is subluxated backward while the radial epiphysis appear to point outward toward the inner third, where an early fusion with the diaphysis occurs.

The deformity is usually bilateral, more common in females, and appears first time in adolescence. The hand and wrist are weak and while wrist flexion is increased, other movements are decreased and painful.

It has been suggested to be a localized chondro-osteodystrophy similar to coxa vara.

Clinical Features

The wrist appears enlarged and dorsiflexion of the hand is impaired. In more severe cases, even supination and pronation are affected. The wrist is loose and insecure and irritable. In long-standing cases, the lower extremity of the radius is bent or curved forward. Pressure on the ulna reduces the deformity which immediately recurs when the pressure is released, owing to laxity of the ligaments of the lower radio-ulnar joint.

Treatment

In recent or acute cases, dorsiflexion of the wrist, maintained by a short plaster case along with a pressure pad over the head of the ulna, gives good results, and care is taken to make sure that the plaster does not interfere with movements at the metacarpophalangeal joints.

In cases of longer standing, an operation is considered.

An osteotomy of the radius has been recommended by some when the articular surface is rotated backward into its normal position and this corrected position is maintained by a plaster cast.

An alternative to this operation is a simpler operation of subperiosteal resection of the distal ulna, which gives satisfactory results.

Dislocated Head of Radius

This condition may be congenital or may follow the failure to reduce a pronation injury, when the patient may notice a lump which is readily palpable and can be felt to move when the forearm is rotated.

Radiographs may reveal the dislocation as congenital, and the radial head may be anterior or posterior when the forearm is rotated. If it is part of a Monteggia fracture dislocation, the forward curve of the mal-united ulna can be seen. If the lump limits elbow flexion, it normally limits elbow flexion and can be excised.

Congenital subluxation of the radial head is usually lateral and is commonly associated with a wide variety of bone dysplasias.

Both elbows may be involved in rheumatoid arthritis, other causes being arthrogryposis multiplex congenita and ankylosing spondylitis. If both the elbows are stiff at impractical angles and the disability is severe, then arthroplasty of one joint can be considered, as one hand is required to reach the mouth.

Congenital synostosis of the superior radio-ulnar joint, along with loss of rotation, is only barely inconvenient, but if the humerus is also involved in the synostosis, then the disability is severe.

Chapter 5
The Wrist Joint

K. Mohan Iyer and Naresh Shetty

Carpal Tunnel Syndrome

Introduction

Carpal tunnel syndrome (CTS) is the most commonly diagnosed and treated entrapment neuropathy. The syndrome is characterized by pain, paresthesia, and weakness in the median nerve distribution of the hand. Surgical and nonsurgical treatments exist that can produce excellent outcomes for patients.

Etiology

The etiology of CTS is multi-factorial, with local and systemic factors contributing to varying degrees. Symptoms of CTS are a result of median nerve compression at the wrist, with ischemia and impaired axonal transport of the median nerve across the wrist. Compression results from elevated pressures within the carpal canal.

Direct pressure or a space-occupying lesion within the carpal canal can increase pressure on the median nerve and produce CTS. Fracture callus, osteophytes, anomalous muscle bodies, tumors, hypertrophic synovium, and infection, as well as gout

K.M. Iyer (✉)
Consultant Orthopedic Surgeon, Bangalore University,
152, Kailash Apartments 8th Main, Malleswaram 120/H-2K,
560 003 Bangalore, Karnataka, India
e-mail: kmiyer28@hotmail.com

N. Shetty, M.S.Orth
Department of Orthopedics, M.S. Ramaiah Medical Teaching Hospital,
Bangalore, Karnataka, 560 054, India

K.M. Iyer (ed.), *Orthopedics of the Upper and Lower Limb*,
DOI 10.1007/978-1-4471-4447-2_5, © Springer-Verlag London 2013

and other inflammatory conditions, can produce increased pressure within the carpal canal. Extremes of wrist flexion and extension also elevate pressure within the carpal canal.

Many systemic conditions are strongly associated with CTS. Individuals with diabetes and hypothyroidism and in women, who are pregnant, are linked to CTS. Conditions affecting metabolism (e.g., alcoholism, renal failure with hemodialysis, mucopolysaccharidosis) also are associated with CTS. Occupational risk factors — repetitive tasks, force, posture, and vibration — have been cited. Psychosocial and socioeconomic issues are increasingly being studied in a study of risk factors for CTS in women.

Pathophysiology

The pathophysiology of CTS is typically demyelination. In more severe cases, secondary axonal loss may be present. The most consistent findings in biopsy specimens of tenosynovium from patients undergoing surgery for idiopathic CTS have been vascular sclerosis and edema.

Clinical Presentation

Acute CTS can develop following a major trauma to the upper extremity (typically a distal radius fracture), a carpal dislocation, or a crush injury. Swelling, pain, and paresthesia in the median nerve distribution of the hand are observed.

In the more common idiopathic or chronic CTS, symptoms are more gradual in onset. Pain and paresthesia in the median nerve distribution of the hand are common. Symptoms are often worse at night and can wake a patient from sleep. As the condition worsens, daytime paresthesia becomes common and is often aggravated by daily activities, such as driving, combing the hair, and holding a book or phone. Weakness can be present. With long-standing or severe cases of CTS, thenar atrophy is frequently observed. Pain and paresthesia can also occur proximally in the forearm, elbow, shoulder, and neck in up to one-third of patients.

Frequency

CTS is common in the general population. It has previously been reported with acute onset following trauma to the wrist. It has also been detailed as a gradual progression of symptoms typically occurring in women who are in the late middle-aged years of life. A new population at risk has been reported to be industrial workers whose hands and wrists are subjected to repetitive motion and trauma.

Investigation

Imaging Studies

- Radiographs
  Patients with a history of systemic disorders, wrist trauma, arthritis, or abnormal findings (e.g., limited motion) on physical examination for CTS are much more likely to have radiographic findings. It is otherwise of limited value.

Other Tests

- Provocative tests.
  - Phalen wrist flexion test – The patient's elbows are placed on a table, with the forearms perpendicular to the table and the wrists flexed. This position is held for 60 s. The test is positive if numbness or paresthesia develops in radial-sided digits.
  - Tinel test – The examiner taps along the course of the median nerve on the volar aspect of the wrist. The test is positive if paresthesia is elicited in the median nerve distribution.
  - Carpal compression test – Direct application of pressure of 150 mmHg or even pressure from both thumbs of the examiner is exerted on the patient's carpal canal and is maintained for 30 s. The test is positive if pain, numbness, or paresthesia develops in the radial-sided digits.
  - Electrophysiologic diagnostic studies – Nerve conduction of median motor and sensory latencies, as well as conduction velocities, are measured across the wrist. A sensory latency of greater than 3.5 ms or a motor latency of greater than 4.5 ms is considered an abnormal finding. Comparison with the contralateral hand, as well as with ulnar motor and sensory latencies and conduction velocities, can provide additional evidence supporting the diagnosis of CTS.

Diagnostic Procedures

- Direct pressure measurement
  - A catheter is inserted directly into the carpal canal to measure pressure.
  - This test is typically used to evaluate acute CTS and can help to differentiate between median nerve contusion and compression.
  - The figure of 30 mmHg is a guide used to determine if the pressure is critically elevated, but physical examination and patient-specific factors can modify the critical pressure.

Treatment

Medical Therapy

Steroid injection and wrist splinting have been used effectively in patients with milder symptoms of CTS. A study reported complete relief of all symptoms in 76 % of hands at 6 weeks after treatment. Similar positive results have been reported with steroid injection. Other nonoperative treatments include non-steroidal anti-inflammatory drugs (NSAIDs).

Surgical Therapy

Open and endoscopic surgical techniques have been described for treatment of CTS. Both operative techniques are effective for the treatment of chronic CTS.

Indications

Acute CTS can be thought of as a compartment syndrome of the carpal canal, and decompression should be performed as soon as possible. Acute CTS can be diagnosed through history and physical examination alone. Electrophysiologic studies are not required. Sometimes, carpal canal pressure measurements are made to help support the diagnosis of acute CTS, with pressures greater than 30 mmHg being consistent with the diagnosis.

Chronic CTS presents over time and is treated in an operative and nonoperative fashion. Patients with milder symptoms and shorter nerve conduction delays on electrodiagnostic studies respond most favorably to nonoperative treatments. Patients with more severe symptoms – duration longer than 1 year, weakness, atrophy, and longer nerve conduction delays – often do not benefit from nonoperative care.

Relevant Anatomy

The carpal canal is a fibro-osseous tunnel at the wrist through which nine flexor tendons and the median nerve pass. The carpal bones define the dorsal aspect of the carpal canal and are shaped in a concave arch. The palmar aspect of the carpal canal is defined by the TCL, which bridges the two sides of the carpal arch. Intrinsic and extrinsic ligaments of the wrist and hand further stabilize the carpal bones. The carpal canal is narrowest at the level of the hook of the hamate, where the canal averages 20 mm in width.

History of the Procedure

In 1854, Sir James Paget first reported median nerve compression at the wrist following a distal radius fracture. In 1913, Pierre Marie and Charles Foix described the pathology of median nerve compression underneath the transverse carpal ligament. In 1933, Sir James Learmonth reported the first TCL release to treat median nerve compression at the wrist. Since these early reports, much work has described the signs and symptoms of CTS, as well as its treatments.

Contraindications

No specific contraindications exist for surgical treatment of CTS. Medical conditions should be stabilized prior to surgery. Pregnancy should be allowed to proceed to term, because CTS often resolves after the pregnancy. Individuals with severe CTS should be cautioned that their numbness may persist, at least to some degree, despite a complete surgical release.

Complications

Complications are not common following open or endoscopic surgical techniques. Major complications with either technique can include nerve laceration, vessel laceration, and tendon laceration. Laceration of the palmar cutaneous branch of the median nerve with painful neuroma formation is reported to be the most common complication of open carpal tunnel release.

Outcome and Prognosis

Lasting relief of pain, numbness, and paresthesia can be expected in more than 90 % of patients with CTS who are treated with open or endoscopic carpal tunnel release; patient satisfaction is high. The primary reason for a poor result is an error in diagnosis.

Future and Controversies

The etiology of CTS and its relationship to the workplace will continue to be better understood in the coming decades. It is already apparent that the etiology of CTS is multifactorial, and although work-induced, repetitive trauma may not be the major cause of CTS, it may contribute in some way.

A realized goal of the less invasive endoscopic technique is to return individuals to work sooner. However, concerns over safety and cost have prevented endoscopic techniques from being widely accepted and used. It is hoped that in the future safer endoscopic methods and less invasive or nonoperative techniques that provide safe and lasting treatment for CTS will be developed.

DeQuervain's Tenosynovitis

- *Stenosing tenosynovitis of first dorsal compartment*: The tendons involved are abductor pollicis longus (APL) and extensor pollicis brevis (EPB). It is seen commonly in 30–50 year olds. It is ten times more common in women and is frequently bilateral.
- Pain with thumb motion over radial styloid. Pain is often felt especially when grasping object then turning the object such as opening a doorknob or turning the ignition key in your car.

It is usually caused by repetitive injury to the hand and arm.

This disorder results when the tendon and its covering (tenosynovium) become inflamed.

- At the wrist and in the palm, tendons glide beneath a system of ligaments and pulleys in a tunnel that increases their mechanical efficiency.
- Where the tendons cross joints, they are sheathed in thin membranes known as synovium, which provide lubrication to decrease friction.

This inflammation can lead to swelling, which further hampers the smooth gliding action of the tendons within the tunnel.

Clinical Findings

- Pain over radial styloid
- Finkelstein's maneuver

DeQuervain's: Treatment

Conservative

- NSAIDs
- Thumb spica splint
- Local Injection of steroids who have not improved with above treatment.

Surgical Management

Operative release required in 25 % of patients after 6 weeks of failed conservative treatment.

Chapter 6
The Hand and Fingers

Shabih Siddiqui

Dupuytren's Contracture

No medical student can escape without being asked about who Dupuytren was!

Baron Dupuytren accurately described the condition in a dissected cadaver hand and presented a detailed account in a paper in 1831. Sir Astley Cooper had earlier described the condition in 1822.

The ring and little finger and ulnar half of the palm is most commonly involved (Fig. 6.1).

Flexion contracture of the fingers, web space contractures, hard and painful nodules in the palm and gradual disuse of the hand and fingers develop slowly over the years. There is extensive fibromatosis of the palmar aponeurosis of the hand.

Dupuytren diathesis involves knuckle pads on the dorsum of the fingers, plantar fibromatosis of the sole of foot and contractures of the penis also called Peyronie's disease.

The main anatomic structures involved are the longitudinal pretendinous bands, the spiral bands, and the natatory ligaments. The lateral digital sheaths, Grayson's ligaments, and the Cleland's ligaments. As these contractures increase fine motor skills, grasp and pinch is affected. Initially the contractures can be passively corrected but as time goes on these contractures become fixed. Later involvement of the muscle and fascia of abductor digiti minimi can contract the little finger further.

Meyerding first described the histologic features in the 1940s. Since then enormous work has been done by several workers explaining the histology and the three main stages have been identified. The initial stage, which is the proliferative stage, involves increase in the cellularity of the palmar fascia.

S. Siddiqui, M.S.Orth, FRCS.Orth
Consultant Orthopedic Surgeon, Kettering General Hospital,
Kettering, UK
e-mail: shabih.s@hotmail.com

K.M. Iyer (ed.), *Orthopedics of the Upper and Lower Limb*,
DOI 10.1007/978-1-4471-4447-2_6, © Springer-Verlag London 2013

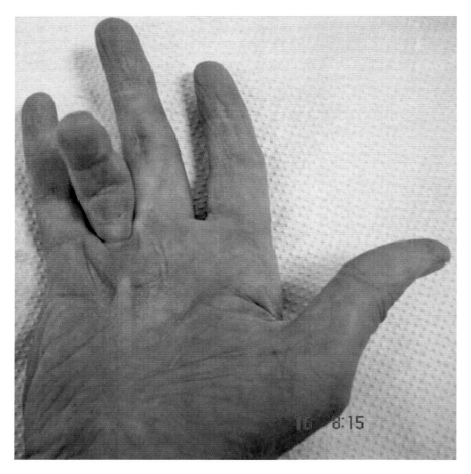

Fig. 6.1 Clinical photograph of Duputren's contracture involving the right ring finger (Courtesy: Dilip Malhotra, Bahrain) (Reproduced with kind permission of Springer Verlag)

The second is the involutional stage in which there is dense myofibroblasts network and less cellular collagen bundles. In the last or residual stage, most myofibroblasts have disappeared and few fibroblasts remain within dense collagen cord.

Dupuytren's disease is more commonly seen in Northern Europe. Non-Caucasians are rarely affected. There is strong association with conditions such as repetitive hand trauma, epilepsy, diabetes mellitus, chronic alcoholism, and chronic lung disease including tuberculosis. It is ten times more common in men than women.

Early treatment may include splinting, steroid use, and physical therapy. Inevitably surgical release is needed. Surgical principles are removal or debulking of contracted palmar fascia, preserving the neurovascular structures, correction of joint deformities, and aggressive physical therapy. Surgery is not curative but can salvage hand function significantly.

A tabletop test in which the hand is held flat on the table and if the palm cannot be kept flat is an indication for surgery. If there is MCP contracture of more than 30°or significant PIP contracture, then surgery is indicated.

Operative procedures include fasciotomy, limited fasciotomy, local fasciotomy, and total radical fasciectomy.

Fasciotomy can be considered for a single contracted palmar band only in experienced hands, as there is risk of damage to neurovascular structures. Total fasciectomy is rarely done due to high morbidity associated with it. Dermo fasciectomy with skin grafting is also done. This has the best chance of preventing recurrence.

Numerous incisions have been used. Skoog and McCash advocate transverse incisions as skin infection and hematoma chances are minimal. Zig Zag incisions and combinations of longitudinal and oblique incisions have been used. Patients are counseled regarding infection, damage to neurovascular structures, and 20–30 % chance of recurrence.

Trigger Finger

Trigger finger – or stenosing tenosynovitis – is a common problem that interferes with the normal function of the fingers or thumbs. This usually affects the middle or ring finger.

It occurs when any digit of the hand gets stuck in a bent or flexed position and causes locking or catching. Overcoming this resistance results in the affected digit snapping straight. If the condition worsens, the finger may need to be forcibly straightened or may remain locked in a bent position.

Causes and Risk Factors

The tendon sheath passes through a canal, which is the A1 pulley at the level of distal crease of the palm.

Trigger finger arises when a nodule, or knot, develops in one of the tendons at this site. Inflammation or scarring is believed to be responsible and is usually the result of repetitive use of the tendon in repeated gripping actions, or an inflammatory condition such as rheumatoid arthritis. There is disparity between the tendon sheath size and the canal through which it passes; hence, the problem is mainly mechanical.

It is more likely to arise in people with medical conditions such as gout and diabetes. However, sometimes there is no explanation why a nodule has developed.

Diagnosis depends entirely on the history and clinical examination. Triggering may be more pronounced in the morning.

Treatment

As the problem is mainly mechanical to overcome trigger finger, any obstruction to normal tendon movement needs to be removed. Specific treatment depends on how severe the symptoms are and how it is affecting an individual.

Mild symptoms may only need the hand to be rested and for repetitive use of the finger to be avoided.

In more serious cases, anti-inflammatory drugs or a steroid injection into the affected tendon should solve the problem.

If these measures are not successful, surgical release, which means releasing the A1 pulley to remove the problematic narrowing, will be recommended. This is usually done as a day case under local anesthesia.

One recent study in the *Journal of Hand Surgery* suggests that the most cost-effective treatment is two trials of corticosteroid injection, followed by open release of the first annular pulley. Choosing surgery immediately is the most expensive option and is often not necessary for resolution of symptoms.

Active and passive physiotherapy will be needed subsequently.

Chapter 7
The Thumb

Shabih Siddiqui

Trigger Thumb in Children (Pediatric Trigger Thumb)

The problem of triggering in children occurs usually in the thumb. It may be noticed soon after birth; hence, it is also sometimes called congenital trigger thumb but a better diagnosis would be pediatric trigger thumb. In adults, it may accompany rheumatoid arthritis.

Children with trigger thumb rarely complain of pain. They are usually brought in for evaluation when aged 1–4 years, when the parent first notices a flexed posture of the thumb IP joint. These children often demonstrate bilateral fixed flexion contractures of the thumb by the time they present to the physician. The diagnosis is made instantaneously as the appearance is classical. One is unable to passively straighten the fixed contracted thumb. A nodule can be felt at the stenosed site.

The cause of trigger thumb is the same as in the finger. There is mechanical obstruction of the tendon of flexor pollicis longus through tight A1 pulley. Apart from being congenital, there may be an element of unnoticed trauma.

Treatment is usually surgical but one must not always rush into surgery as in some studies there is spontaneous recovery in 30 % cases. Recovery is unlikely if the child is more than 2 years.

In children, the procedure is performed under a general anesthetic under a tourniquet. A transverse or curvilinear incision centered over the MCP joint of the thumb was made on the volar aspect. This is centered over the nodule. The A1 pulley is cleanly divided longitudinally. The tendon of the FPL is then delivered in the wound with a curved hemostat. The edges of the pulley may be excised. Full excursion of the thumb is then observed to make sure no secondary adhesions are present. It is obvious to say that the neurovascular structures are protected. Skin is closed with absorbable sutures and thumb movements are encouraged as soon as possible.

S. Siddiqui, M.S.Orth, FRCS.Orth
Consultant Orthopedic Surgeon, Kettering General Hospital, Kettering, UK
e-mail: shabih.s@hotmail.com

K.M. Iyer (ed.), *Orthopedics of the Upper and Lower Limb*,
DOI 10.1007/978-1-4471-4447-2_7, © Springer-Verlag London 2013

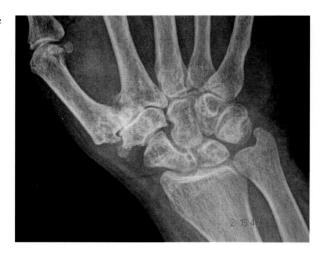

Fig. 7.1 Osteoarthritis of the carpometacarpal joint of the thumb (Courtesy: Dilip Malhotra, Bahrain)

Osteoarthritis of Thumb

This condition is seen fairly common in those who have done a heavy physical job but can also present in the general population especially females. The carpometa-carpal joint is involved: the trapezium being commonly involved and sometimes the trapezium trapezoid complex is involved as a whole. Previous trauma can also cause secondary OA at this joint. Patients with rheumatoid disease commonly have some degree of involvement of this joint.

There may in addition be osteoarthritis of the proximal and distal interphalangeal joints with Herbeden and Bouchard's nodes.

Physical examination reveals pain, tenderness, and swelling at the joint site. There is reduction of joint movement. The grind and circumduction tests reveal sharp pain. Crepitus is fairly common.

Painful instability of the carpometacarpal joint is frequently seen. The scaphora-dial joint may frequently be involved.

X-rays confirm the diagnosis (Fig. 7.1) and no more sophisticated tests are needed.

Early osteoarthritis of the thumb is treated conservatively by nonsteroidal agents and splinting. Physical therapy can sometimes produce dramatic improvement. Steroid injections are frequently given in outpatients followed by hand therapy.

Surgery is reserved for those cases that fail medical management.

Fusion of CMC joint is a viable option for younger patients who do not want to risk loss of strength, which is inevitable after joint arthroplasty. Relief of pain is good but fine motor function may be compromised.

Joint Arthroplasty

Plastic or metal prosthesis is used to replace the worn-out joints. This is usually done for elderly or rheumatoid patients. This can also be done after failed arthrodesis.

Chapter 8
Hand Infections

Shabih Siddiqui

With the advent of strong antibiotics, the sequelae of threatening infections of the hand are rarely to be seen these days. Early recognition, adequate and aggressive surgical intervention, and methodical timely rehabilitation have been responsible for a favorable outcome in the majority of infections.

The hand is expected to perform beyond expectations: From day to day activities, to be the breadwinner, and even to perform magic, such are the expectations of the hand. Untreated hand infections can lead such a vital and dexterous organ to turn out into a painful and useless appendage.

Paronychia

Paronychia is the most common infection of the hand. Commonly caused by foreign material implantation or by hangnail. The infection starts as a subcuticular abscess in the paronychial fold (Fig. 8.1) Causation is by both aerobic and anaerobic bacterial flora. Common organisms are *Staph aureus*, group A streptococci, bacteroids, etc.

Initial treatment is by warm soaks, spitting, and antibiotics. Incision and drainage is needed if simple treatment fails. Part of nail may have to be removed to completely decompress. Augmentin is commonly used to treat the infection.

S. Siddiqui, M.S.Orth, FRCS.Orth
Consultant Orthopedic Surgeon, Kettering General Hospital,
Kettering, UK
e-mail: shabih.s@hotmail.com

K.M. Iyer (ed.), *Orthopedics of the Upper and Lower Limb*,
DOI 10.1007/978-1-4471-4447-2_8, © Springer-Verlag London 2013

Fig. 8.1 Clinical photograph
of paronychia (Courtesy:
Shabih Siddiqui, Kettering,
UK) (Reproduced with kind
permission of Springer
Verlag)

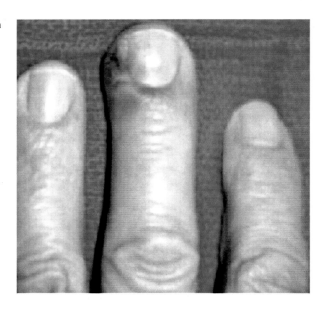

Felon

A felon is an abscess of the terminal pulp space of the phalanx. There are 15–20
septa running from the periosteum to skin of distal phalanx. This explains why these
closed space abscesses are so painful and if not treated adequately may cause osteomyelitis of the phalanx. Commonly caused by puncture wounds or foreign bodies
and the causative organisms are same as for paronychia.

Initially there is cellulitis, swelling, and tenderness(Fig. 8.2). Untreated abscess
can form rapidly. Complications include osteomyelitis, flexor tenosynovitis, or pyogenic arthritis of the terminal joint leading to long-term stiffness and pain.

Early treatment includes warm soaks, antibiotics, and limb elevation and if not
successful incision and drainage is resorted to.

A longitudinal incision or a classic hockey stick incision is given and all septae
are knocked down.

Tendon Sheath Infections

Once again these are the result of foreign body implantation, puncture wounds, or
lacerations. Prompt identification and treatment is mandatory as infection can rapidly spread proximally, may cause destruction of pulley system or tendon absorption. History and Kanavel's four classic signs clinch diagnosis: tenderness over the
involved tendon sheath, pain on passive extension of finger, fusiform swelling of
finger, and flexed attitude of finger.

Fig. 8.2 Clinical photograph
of pulp infection (Courtesy:
Shabih Siddiqui, Kettering,
UK) (Reproduced with kind
permission of Springer
Verlag)

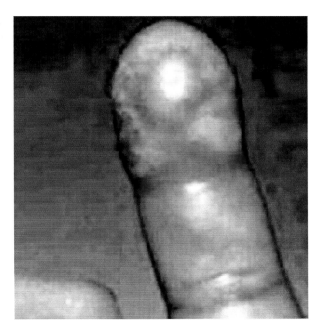

The index, middle, and the ring fingers are commonly involved. Coagulase positive *Staph aureus* is commonly involved but gram-negative organisms are also frequently involved. Early antibiotic therapy may be curative but if after 24–36 h infection is not subsiding incision and drainage should be performed. Closed irrigation with a fine catheter may be done along with parenteral antibiotics.

Thenar and Midpalmar Infections

These are two potential closed spaces of the hand. The boundaries of the thenar space are as follows: on the ulnar side by the midpalmar oblique septum, volarly by index finger profundus tendon, and on the dorsal side by the adductor pollicis.

Infections in this area present with marked pain, swelling tenderness, and pushing the thumb into abduction.

The midpalmar space is bounded dorsally by the third, fourth, and the fifth metacarpals, volarly by the flexor tendons, radially by the midpalmar septum, and ulnarly by the hypothenar septum.

Proximally these spaces are till the distal limit of the carpal tunnel.

Midpalmar space infections present with swelling not only in the palm but also dorsally. Fluctuation, erythema, and tenderness are however more in the palm. Motion of the middle, ring, and little fingers is reduced.

Treatment of thenar and midpalmar space infections is incision and drainage. Initially broad-spectrum antibiotics are started followed by culture-specific antibiotics.

Herpetic Whitlow

This is a viral infection of the fingers caused by contact with herpes simplex virus. Predominantly seen in health care workers because of their frequent contact with oral and genital secretions of patients. Incubation period varies between 2 and 20 days. There is intense throbbing pain and erythema. Vesicles filled with clear fluid, which might coalesce to from bulla. Treatment is usually symptomatic and Acyclovir may be reserved for severe cases. Surgical drainage can lead to disastrous complications, hence important to distinguish this condition from paronychia, etc.

Human and Animal Bites

Any doctor working in the A&E department knows how frequently these injuries are especially on a Saturday night. Apart from human bites, dog and cat bites are common. There is a mixture of inoculating organisms and some of the serious sequelae are osteomyelitis, chronic stiffness of finger, amputation, and even death. Tetanus and rabies must always be at the back of the mind of the treating physician.

These wounds need early and thorough irrigation and must be left open. They are secondarily closed if needed.

The common causative organisms include *Streptococcus*, *Staph aureus*, and *Pasteurella multocida*. These organisms are susceptible to a variety of antibiotics, and help from the microbiology department is well worth the effort.

Human bites commonly cause penetration of the metacarpophalangeal joint especially if assault is the mechanism of injury. Once again thorough exploration and irrigation is needed along with appropriate antibiotics which initially are parenteral and subsequently oral.

Necrotizing Fasciitis

This is a particularly extremely dangerous condition the incidence of which has been substantially increased in the last 20 years.

It can be potentially limb and life threatening. It is a soft tissue infection manifested by rapidly progressive inflammation and necrosis of subcutaneous fat, fascia, skin, and muscle.

The most common organism involved is Group A *Streptococcus*. An early diagnosis and high index of suspicion is the key to success. Patients with reduced host defenses are particularly liable to infection.

Early and radical surgical debridement with ruthless removal of necrotic tissue is the key to successful salvage of limb and life. Patients need judicious use of antibiotics as well as intravenous resuscitation and medical support.

Tuberculous Infection of Hand

The infection may begin in the tenosynovium of the long flexor tendons of the hand and may be the only manifestation of the disease. It may spread to adjacent bones and joints. Metacarpals can be involved causing tuberculous dactylitis. Differential diagnosis includes rheumatoid arthritis, synovitis, sarcoidosis non-specific synovitis, and fungal infections.

A biopsy may show AFB or caseating granulomas with Langham giant cells. Tuberculosis of wrist may present as Carpal Tunnel Syndrome. Rice bodies may be found during Carpal Tunnel Release. Treatment includes synovial biopsy, surgical debridement, and multi-therapy antituberculous drugs.

Part II
The Lower Limb

Chapter 9
The Hip Joint

Dipen K. Menon

Introduction

The hip is a ball and socket joint with considerable freedom of movement. Loss of hip movement can be compensated by pelvic and spinal movement. Hip deformity can be masked by compensation in the lumbar spine and pelvis. This forms the basis of the Thomas' test (see below). Pelvic movement has to be eliminated to test true movement in the hip. The hip can be affected by a multitude of conditions and forms the basis of this chapter. Hip fractures, which would fall under the category of Trauma, will be dealt with in a separate section.

Symptoms

Hip Pain

Patients usually complain of pain in the groin which radiates to the front of the thigh, extending down to the knee. Patients may also complain of pain in the buttock and over the flare of the greater trochanter. Occasionally patients with hip disease may present with pain solely in the ipsilateral knee area. This can lead to misdiagnosis and occasionally result in the misdirection of treatment to the uninvolved knee. Hip pain like other lower limb joint pains is usually aggravated by weight

D.K. Menon, MS Orth (AIIMS), DNB (Orth), MCh (Orth) Liverpool, FRCS (Tr & Orth)
Department of Consultant Orthopedic Surgeon, University of Leicester,
Leicester, UK

Kettering General Hospital,
Rothwell Road, Kettering, Northamptonshire NN16 8UZ, UK
e-mail: dipenmenon@aol.com

K.M. Iyer (ed.), *Orthopedics of the Upper and Lower Limb*,
DOI 10.1007/978-1-4471-4447-2_9, © Springer-Verlag London 2013

bearing and progressively restricts the ability of patients to ambulate. Pain occurring during rest usually signifies more advanced hip disease. Patients also experience difficulty in sleeping and finding a position of comfort in bed. This may result from increased local pressure over the painful area or from relaxation of muscle spasm during sleep causing the patient to awake. The sleep can be particularly affected in patients with bilateral hip disease. Analgesics and anti-inflammatories may help relieve pain, particularly in inflammatory conditions.

Limp

Patients can limp from of a variety of reasons. Pain can result in an antalgic gait (stance phase on affected limb shortened to reduce the pain produced by weight bearing). Hip stiffness can result in a stiff hip gait where the pelvis and spine move during the swing phase to compensate for the lack of hip movement. Functional shortening or lengthening can result in dipping and vaulting type of gait patterns, respectively. Abductor weakness can result in a Trendelenburg gait where the pelvis sags on the side of the unaffected hip when weight bearing on the affected leg. This loss of balance is compensated for by an upper body and shoulder tilt toward the side of the affected hip. Patients may use a walking-stick to off-load the affected hip.

Deformity

Hip deformity can be masked by the lumbar spine and the pelvis. The examiner requires to unravel this to actually define the hip deformity. Rotational deformity cannot be masked by the pelvis and is therefore easily visible even to the untrained eye.

Swelling

The hip is a deep-seated joint and is well covered with muscles. Swellings in and around the hip are usually not visible because of this. Advanced tumors or a psoas abscess may manifest as a visible swelling in the groin or buttock.

Stiffness

Hip stiffness after a period of inactivity occurs as a result of capsular inflammation and fibrosis. Patients may complain of difficulty in getting out of a chair. This may be associated with a start-up type of pain and stiffness which settles after a variable period of walking. Patients may also complain of difficulty in donning and doffing their shoes and socks or cutting their toe-nails as a result of hip stiffness.

Signs

It is important to gather visual cues right from the time patients walk in for their consultation. The manner in which the patient dresses and undresses can also provide the examiner with very useful information. The usual system of examination is followed to avoid missing important findings. This system incorporates the logically progressive steps: look, feel, move, and measure (Apley).

Look

Looking begins right from the time the patient comes into the consultation room. This would include noticing if the patient walks with a limp, uses a shoe raise or a walking-stick. Patients find ways around removing their trousers, shoes, and socks when the hip is stiff. This could include standing with the hip extended, knee fully flexed, and taking the hand behind the back to pull the shoes off for example. Patients may opt to wear slip-on shoes to avoid tying their shoe laces. On removing the clothes, muscle wasting becomes obvious if one compares the two legs from the front, the sides, and the back. Discharging sinuses or puckered scars may suggest an ongoing or a previous infection, respectively. Surgical scars would indicate the approach used for previous surgery on the hip. Asymmetric creases on the medial side of the thigh are important in infants and young children to diagnose hip dislocation. An external rotation deformity (foot facing outward) is visible if one compares this with the foot on the normal unaffected hip. Observing the gait pattern is important (see above).

Feel

Feeling the anatomical landmarks around the hip and tender areas can indicate sources of pain. Tenderness over the greater trochanter may indicate trochanteric bursitis. The precise anatomical structure causing pain can sometimes be difficult to ascertain due to the fact that many of these are deep seated. Feeling anatomical landmarks can help identify shortening above the level of the trochanter suggesting shortening in the hip or the femoral neck. To establish shortening of a limb, it is important to ascertain that the pelvis is square (i.e., that both anterior superior iliac spines are at the same level). As the pelvis compensates for coronal plane deformity of the hip, actual shortening of the leg, and spinal deformity (scoliosis), it is important to differentiate between the three of them. Unless the pelvic obliquity is fixed (i.e., not flexible), sitting down will obliterate the obliquity. Feeling the patient's spinous processes in the sitting position will reveal scoliosis of the spine. True shortening of the leg may become obvious in this position.

Move

Flexion deformity, which is a sagittal plane deformity of the hip, can be masked by forward pelvic tilt resulting in an increase in lumbar lordosis. Flexion deformity can be revealed by performing the Thomas' test. With the patient in the supine position, the lumbar lordosis is obliterated by fully flexing the unaffected hip and knee so that the thigh is brought toward the abdomen. Flexion deformity in the affected hip will be revealed by this maneuver. Further flexion in the hip is measured from this position of deformity. Other movements to be checked are abduction, adduction, internal and external rotation. It is important to stabilize the pelvis by placing the examiner's forearm over the pelvis horizontally when these movements are being tested. The two hips are compared and the range of movement in degrees is recorded.

Measure

The limb can be shortened because of hip disease. This can manifest as true shortening when there is hip joint destruction or subluxation. As shortening can occur in the tibial, femoral, or hip segments of the leg, a useful test is the Galleazzi test (Fig. 9.1) to differentiate between the former two. The two legs are kept in contact at the knees and heels and flexed to 90°. Both heels are placed at the same distance from the buttocks and the height of the legs at the level of the two knees is compared. This test can differentiate between shortening in the tibial and femoral segments of the limb. Any shortening above the trochanter can be ascertained by drawing a line joining the two anterior superior iliac spines (ASIS) and comparing the distance between the tip of the greater trochanter and this line in each limb. True shortening can be measured by squaring the pelvis and measuring the distance between the ASIS and medial malleolus of each leg using a measuring tape.

The leg can be shortened or lengthened due to coronal plane hip deformity and pelvic compensation (apparent shortening or lengthening). An abduction deformity would cause the pelvis to tilt in a downward direction on the side of the affected hip in order to facilitate walking. This would make it look like the opposite limb is short and the affected limb is longer. Likewise with an adduction deformity the pelvis tilts upward on the affected side making the affected limb look shorter than its fellow.

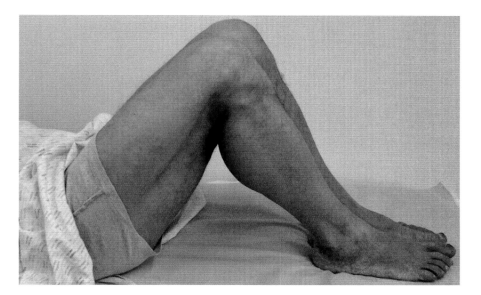

Fig. 9.1 Galleazzi test demonstrating femoral shortening in the right lower limb

Investigations

Bloods

Full blood count, erythrocyte sedimentation rate (ESR), and C-reactive protein (CRP) are helpful in supporting a diagnosis of infective, inflammatory, and neo-plastic conditions. These are termed as acute phase markers. The response to treatment can be monitored by repeating the CRP and studying its trends. The CRP is sensitive and in combination with the ESR can increase specificity in diagnosing and monitoring infection. This is particularly useful in prosthetic infection. The bone profile (serum calcium, phosphate, and alkaline phosphatase) is useful in the diagnosis of metabolic and neoplastic hip conditions. Rheumatoid factor is an auto-antibody which is positive in sero-positive rheumatoid arthritis. Serum electrophoresis and Urine Bence Jones proteins can establish the diagnosis in multiple myeloma.

X-Rays

The usual view required is an antero-posterior view of the pelvis (AP Pelvis) show-ing both hips and sacro-iliac joints. This view can show fractures of the pelvis and

Fig. 9.2 AP pelvic X-ray
showing partial bony
obliteration of both sacro-
iliac joints in ankylosing
spondylitis

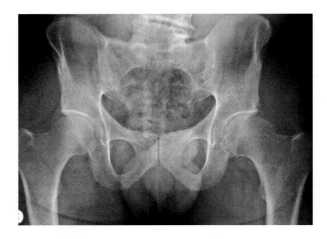

hip joint. Dislocations of the hip can also be diagnosed on this view. By obtaining
an AP Pelvis X-ray, the two hips can be compared and any differences noted. Any
reduction in joint space, particularly in the weight-bearing portion, is suggestive of
osteoarthritis (degenerative joint disease). This can be associated with subchondral
cysts, osteophytes, and sub-chondral bone sclerosis. Avascular necrosis and Perthes'
disease is associated with collapse and alteration in the shape of the femoral head.
A concentric reduction in joint space is suggestive of an inflammatory arthritis.
Obliteration of the sacro-iliac joints or any destruction around these joints can be
suggestive of ankylosing spondylitis (Fig. 9.2) or an infective process like tuberculosis. A lateral view of the affected hip can also show a reduction in joint space
suggestive of osteoarthritis. Fractures and slipped capital femoral epiphysis can be
diagnosed on this view.

Arthrography

This is performed by injecting iodine containing contrast into the hip and taking an
X-ray. The hip can be moved and screened under X-ray (Image intensifier) control.
This can therefore be a dynamic investigation. This is particularly useful in decision
making in dysplastic conditions of the hip and Perthes' disease.

Ultrasound Scan

Ultrasound scans are non-invasive and can show a hip effusion and fluid collections
around the hip. This can be helpful in diagnosing septic arthritis in the presence of
other clinical features. It is also a very useful screening investigation in diagnosing
congenital hip dislocation.

Bone Scan

This is performed by injecting a radioactive compound containing either technetium, gallium, or indium and then taking images using a gamma camera. This is
helpful in diagnosing bone and soft-tissue infection, tumors (particularly meta-
static), and assessing alterations in blood supply to the femoral head.

CT Scan (Computerized Axial Tomography)

CT scans show bone architecture well and can help show the morphology of fractures of the pelvis, acetabulum, and hip joint. CT scans are helpful in preoperative
planning. Modern scanners can show sagittal reconstructions and three-dimensional
re-formatted scans of the area of interest.

MRI Scan (Magnetic Resonance Imaging)

MRI scans can reveal bone and soft-tissue detail with considerable clarity. Areas
of edema and alterations in blood supply can be visualized. This is a particularly
helpful investigation in diagnosing and grading avascular necrosis of the hip.
This is also used routinely in the grading and staging of primary bone and soft-
tissue tumors around the hip and in the pelvis. This is an expensive investigation
and is only very occasionally required in the management of routine hip
problems.

Developmental Dysplasia of the Hip

Developmental dysplasia represents a spectrum of conditions affecting the hip. At
the most extreme end of this spectrum is congenital hip dislocation. It affects the
newborn child (Figs. 9.3 and 9.4).

   In utero the hip and knees are held in a flexed position with both ankles dorsiflexed.
This position helps in keeping the fetus compact occupying minimum volume
within the uterus. The hips remain flexed at birth and progressively extend in
infancy.

   Congenital dislocation of the hip affects about 1–2 in a 1,000 infants. It is
more common in girls. There is a genetic predisposition to develop this condition. It is more common in the breech presentation where the hips are held in
extension in utero.

Fig. 9.3 Developmental
dysplasia of the hip
(Courtesy: Magdi E. Greiss,
Whitehaven, Cumbria, UK)

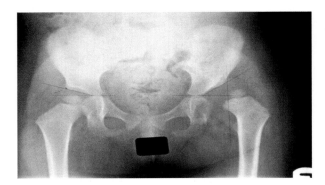

Fig. 9.4 Developmental
dysplasia, treated by
derotational osteotomy of the
femur (Courtesy: Magdi E.
Greiss, Whitehaven,
Cumbria, UK)

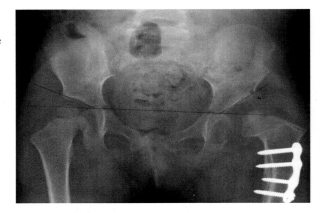

Pathological Anatomy

The direction of dislocation is usually posterior. The acetabulum is shallow and the ligamentum teres is hypertrophied. The acetabular labrum may be inverted. The hypertrophied ligamentum teres and the inverted labrum (limbus) may prevent the closed reduction of a dislocated hip particularly in a late presentation. The capsule is usually lax. Ossification of the femoral capital epiphysis is delayed and acetabular development will also be abnormal.

Clinical Features

The newborn child may have a dislocated hip or an unstable hip. There are two screening tests in the newborn baby.

Ortolani's Test

This test confirms that the dislocated hip is reducible. The newborn is held on the mother's lap or supine. The examiner places the fingers of each hand on the posterior aspect of each hip and the upper thigh with the hips flexed to 90°. The thumbs are placed in front of each hip over the empty acetabulum. A gentle abduction and forward-pushing force is applied with the fingers. The dislocated hip reduces with a clunk.

Barlow's Test

This is a provocative test that confirms that the hip is dislocatable (unstable). The newborn is examined in the same position as above and the hips are held in the same way as for the Ortolani's test. The reduced abducted hips are then adducted with a gentle telescoping force applied in the long axis of the limb. The hip dislocates with a click.

A persistently dislocated hip presents with a lack of abduction. The affected leg is shortened in unilateral hip dislocation and there may be asymmetric skin creases on the medial aspect of the thighs.

Investigations

Ultrasound Scan

Routine screening of all newborns with an ultrasound scan is the norm in certain countries like Austria. In the UK, high-risk newborns are screened, i.e., family history, breech presentation, and in clinically dislocated or dislocatable hips. This is a dynamic investigation and provocative tests can be performed under ultrasound control. Reduction can be confirmed during treatment.

X-Rays

X-rays are useful after the age of 6 months. X-rays can be useful to ascertain the position of the femoral capital epiphysis with respect to the quadrants created by drawing the Hilgenreiner's (horizontal) and Perkins's (vertical) lines (90° to each other) on an AP view of the pelvis (Fig. 9.5). The normal femoral capital epiphysis lies in the infero-medial quadrant. Acetabular development can be assessed by calculating the acetabular index (Fig. 9.6), which is the angle between the acetabular roof line and the Hilgenreiner's line (normal: between 27° and 30° at birth and decreasing to 20° by the age of 2 years). In acetabular dysplasia, this angle is above 30°. The Shenton's line is an arc drawn between the medial border of the femoral neck and the superior border of the obturator foramen. This should be a continuous arc without any disruption in it. A disruption signifies hip dislocation (Fig. 9.7).

Fig. 9.5 Dislocation of the right hip. The femoral capital epiphysis is smaller and located in the upper outer quadrant

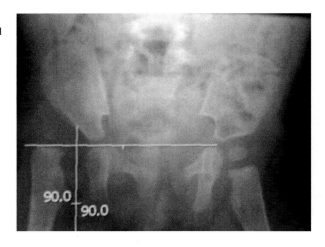

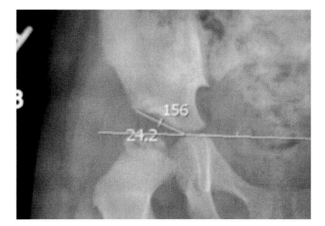

Fig. 9.6 The acetabular index: 24.2°. Angle between the Hilgenreiner's line and acetabular roof line

Fig. 9.7 Anteroposterior radiograph of the pelvis with both hips showing bilateral congenital dislocation of the hip (Courtesy: Dilip Malhotra, Bahrain) (Reproduced with kind permission of Springer Verlag)

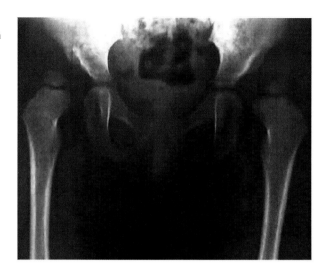

Treatment

Age	Treatment
Birth to 6 months	Closed reduction and Pawlik harness in 90° hip flexion and abduction in the safe zone of Ramsey (remember excessive adduction dislocates and excessive abduction can compromise blood supply to the femoral capital epiphysis resulting in avascular necrosis). Hip reduction has to be gentle. The required flexion and abduction can be achieved by adjusting the straps on the harness
	Child older than 3 months: adductor tenotomy may be necessary
	Duration of harness treatment is between 3 and 9 months on average depending on the age of initiation of harness treatment. Regular monitoring is necessary to confirm that the hip is reduced concentrically
6–18 months	Closed or open reduction and immobilization in a hip spica. An arthrogram may be useful to confirm reduction and to assess if there are any soft-tissue obstructions to closed reduction (e.g., inverted limbus, hypertrophied ligamentum teres). Adductor tenotomy is usually required. Spica treatment may be required for between 6 weeks and 6 months depending on hip stability

Age	Treatment
18 months to 4 years	Open reduction is required and is the safe option. Acetabular development is abnormal and there may be persistent femoral anteversion. Open reduction may therefore require to be combined with a pelvic, e.g., Salter innominate osteotomy and/or a femoral (de-rotation) osteotomy and shortening
Above age of 8 years	Reduction not attempted in unilateral dislocation because of the risk of avascular necrosis resulting in a painful hip. In bilateral hip dislocation, it is better to avoid operation in children above the age of 6 as they adapt well to their deformity
Adult dislocation or hip dysplasia with secondary OA and pain	Total hip replacement (Figs. 9.8 and 9.9). Femoral shortening may be required in addition

Fig. 9.8 Sequelae of CDH in a man aged 58 years (Courtesy: Magdi E. Greiss, Whitehaven, Cumbria, UK)

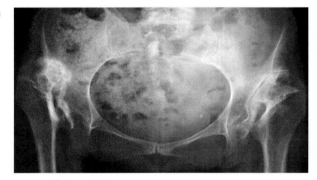

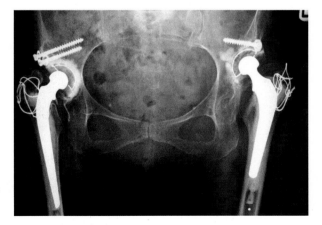

Fig. 9.9 Bilateral total hip replacement done with patient's own femoral heads as grafts (Courtesy: Magdi E. Greiss, Whitehaven, Cumbria, UK)

Fig. 9.10 External rotation of the right hip on flexion in SCFE

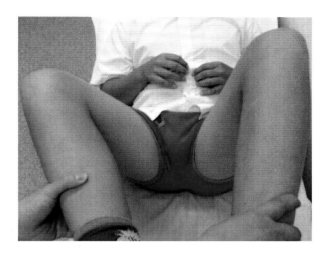

Slipped Capital Femoral Epiphysis

This is a condition that occurs in adolescents during the pubertal growth spurt. It is more common in boys. The (capital) upper femoral epiphysis displaces through the zone of hypertrophy in the physis. The children who slip their femoral epiphysis usually have a higher than normal body mass index. The condition is postulated to occur due to an imbalance between the growth and gonadotrophic hormones. The presentation can be acute (symptomatic for a period less than 3 weeks), chronic (symptomatic for a period more than 3 weeks), or acute on chronic (chronically symptomatic culminating in an acute exacerbation). The condition can occur bilaterally.

Patients usually present with groin or knee pain and a limp. This may follow a traumatic episode and is commonly misdiagnosed as a groin strain. In more severe cases, the child may be unable to weight-bear on the affected leg. On examination there may be shortening and external rotation of the affected leg. Flexing the affected hip will cause the leg to externally rotate in a chronic healed slip (Figs. 9.10 and 9.11). Attempted movement in all directions is painful and associated with muscle spasm.

X-rays may show an obvious slip (Fig. 9.12), although the appearances can sometimes be subtle and missed as a result. On an antero-posterior view a line drawn along the superior margin of the femoral neck passes through the epiphysis (Trethowan's sign). On a lateral view the femoral epiphysis is tilted backward with respect to the axis of the femoral neck (resembling a dollop of ice-cream that has slipped off its cone).

Treatment

In mild and moderate acute slips, the epiphysis is pinned in situ (Figs. 9.13 and 9.14). Manipulation is not attempted in order to preserve the remaining blood supply to the epiphysis. A corrective sub-trochanteric osteotomy can be performed

Fig. 9.11 Shortening and external rotation of the right leg in SCFE

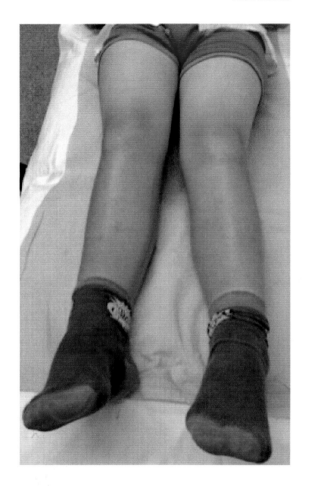

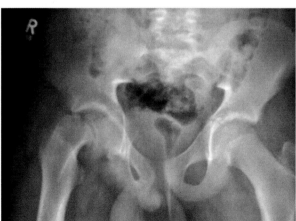

Fig. 9.12 Slipped right capital femoral epiphysis

Fig. 9.13 Anteroposterior radiograph of the pelvis taken in frog's view showing a slipped upper femoral epiphysis on the *left side* (Courtesy: Dilip Malhotra, Bahrain) (Reproduced with kind permission of Springer Verlag)

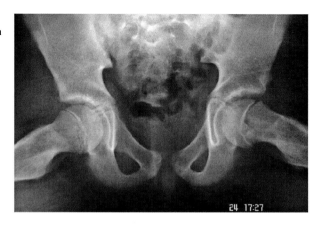

Fig. 9.14 Pinning of SCFE in situ

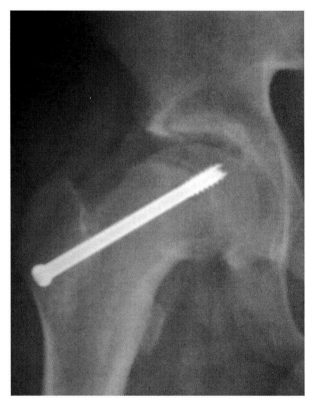

once healing has occurred if there is any significant residual deformity. The aim of treatment is to fix the epiphysis without damaging its blood supply. Any damage to the epiphyseal blood supply would inevitably lead to avascular necrosis. In severe slips, an open reduction maybe necessary before any fixation can be performed.

Septic Arthritis

Infection can affect the hip joint both in children and adults. This condition is more common in the extremes of age and particularly in infants and children. Proteolytic enzymes produced by bacteria can rapidly destroy cartilage and it is therefore imperative to diagnose and treat this condition early to get an optimal result. The predisposition to and the severity of infection depends on host immunity and the virulence of the infecting organism.

Common Infecting Organisms

Staphylococcus
Streptococcus
Pneumococcus
Haemophilus

Clinical Features

Systemic symptoms include fever, malaise, rigors, sweats, loss of appetite and weight. Classic systemic features may not always be present in the extremes of age or if antibiotics have already been administered empirically. The history of a preceding flu or respiratory infection may be forthcoming.

Local symptoms include pain, limp, pseudo-paralysis, and difficulty in weight-bearing on the affected leg. Local tenderness may be elicited in the groin. Attempted passive and active hip movements will be painful and associated with spasm.

Investigations

X-rays may not reveal any abnormality apart from soft-tissue swelling. Ultrasound scanning may reveal an effusion. It is possible to aspirate the effusion in adults under LA and ultrasound guidance. In children, aspiration is better performed under a GA. The treatment of choice is arthrotomy, thorough washout, and closure of the hip. This procedure may require to be repeated again depending on the clinical response. The aspirate should be sent for gram staining and culture and sensitivity studies. Antibiotics should be started as soon as the diagnosis can be established with reasonable certainty. The initial antibiotic prescribed is based on the most likely organism and a microbiologist's advice can be helpful. Antibiotics may require to be continued for approximately 6 weeks and the acute phase markers (full blood count, ESR, and CRP) can help determine when they can be stopped.

Fig. 9.15 Septic arthritis of the hip joint (Courtesy: Magdi E. Greiss, Whitehaven, Cumbria, UK)

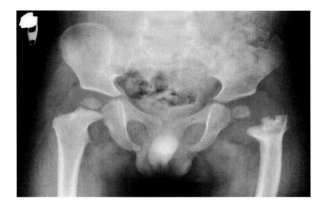

Complications

Septic arthritis, particularly in children, can be associated with destruction of the femoral head which can lead to dislocation or result in a pseudarthrosis. (Tom Smith's arthritis) (Fig. 9.15). In adults, there can be significant hip destruction resulting in stiffness (ankylosis) or secondary osteoarthritis.

Tuberculosis of the Hip

Tuberculous hip joint disease usually progresses from the surrounding subchondral and metaphyseal bone. As the epiphysis and metaphysis are intra-articular, spread of infection into the joint can occur early in the disease process. This then manifests as synovitis, destructive arthritis, and cold abscesses. It can cause significant hip destruction if the diagnosis is delayed. The usual foci of initial involvement are the superior part of the acetabulum, the femoral capital epiphysis, and the medial metaphysis of the hip. The disease process can start in region of the trochanteric bursa and not involve the hip joint at all. The disease usually affects children and young adults.

Diagnosis

Children usually present with groin pain radiating to the knee. This is associated with a limp (antalgic gait) and deformity. Fullness may be seen or felt in the groin as a result of cold abscess formation. The pain may be severe at night, frequently waking and causing distress to the child (night cries). Synovitis is associated with an effusion and the patient holds the hip in the position of ease (flexion, abduction, and external rotation). This causes apparent lengthening of the involved limb (see above). Tenderness maybe elicited by applying local pressure in the groin. As the disease progresses, there is muscle wasting and muscle spasm leading to a flexion adduction and internal rotation deformity. There is true shortening due to a combination of joint destruction and varying degrees of subluxation.

Investigations

The acute phase markers are raised and the Mantoux test is usually positive once the disease is well established (present for more than 6–12 weeks). X-rays in the early stages may not reveal any abnormality or only a small focus of bone destruction. Ultrasound may reveal an effusion, cold abscess, or synovial thickening in the early stages of the disease. Once tuberculous arthritis sets in, destructive changes in the bone and joint become visible. Any fluid aspirate should be sent for AFB staining and culture and sensitivity studies. Tissue biopsy can establish the diagnosis but is not necessary if the diagnosis can be established on clinical grounds.

Treatment

Anti-tuberculous drugs are commenced on making the diagnosis. Traction is useful in relieving muscle spasm and in the prevention of deformity. Cold abscesses can be aspirated. Weight-bearing may have to be commenced based on the extent of joint involvement, bone destruction, and the response to treatment. Surgical debridement is reserved for patients who do not respond to medical treatment. Secondary procedures maybe required once the disease has been eradicated. These include arthrodesis, Girdlestone excision arthroplasty, and total hip replacement (the latter in carefully selected patients).

Meralgia Paraesthetica

This condition occurs due to compression of the lateral cutaneous nerve of the thigh as it runs under the lateral aspect of the inguinal ligament. This can result in neuralgic pain, paraesthesiae, and numbness on the anterolateral aspect of the thigh (L1,2,3 dermatomes) . This pain can be confused with hip pain. It may be possible to reproduce the patient's symptoms by local percussion over the trigger area. Initial treatment with a local steroid injection around the trigger area can sometimes be helpful. In resistant cases, decompression of the lateral cutaneous nerve of the thigh may be required.

Fig. 9.16 Femoral head in OA showing patchy cartilage loss and eburnation (Courtesy: Dipen Menon, Kettering, UK)

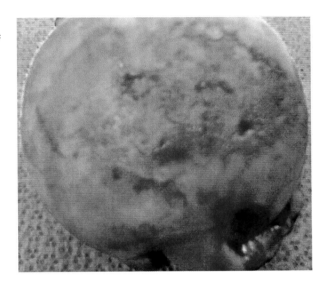

Trochanteric Bursitis

Patients may complain of pain over the trochanteric region. The trochanteric area maybe tender to local palpation. The trochanteric bursa may be inflamed and crepitus maybe elicited in this area. Bursae can be inflamed in gout or inflammatory arthritis. The inflammation may also be as a result of previous surgery to this area (e.g., total hip replacement or fracture fixation). Local physiotherapy to the area can sometimes be helpful. Other treatment options include a local steroid injection once infection has been excluded. In resistant cases, the bursa can be excised or protruding metalwork resulting from fracture fixation removed.

Osteoarthritis (OA)

Osteoarthritis is a disorder where there is softening and progressive destruction of articular cartilage associated with a healing response (Fig. 9.16). Primary OA is usually a disease that affects the older population (over 50 years of age). The term secondary OA is used when there is an underlying cause for arthritis. The usual causes of secondary OA are fractures (particularly intra-articular: involving the joint surface), avascular necrosis, inflammatory arthritis, infection, and acetabular dysplasia. Secondary OA can occur in younger patients. OA has a multifactorial etiology with genetic factors, local trauma, and metabolic factors being implicated. The disease commonly affects weight-bearing joints. The hip joint is commonly affected in primary OA. Local increase in stress in weight-bearing joints in patients with a high body mass index can predispose to the development of OA.

Fig. 9.17 Bilateral OA hips (Courtesy: Dipen Menon, Kettering, UK)

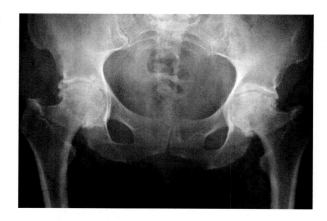

Diagnosis

Patients complain of groin pain on weight-bearing which can progressively restrict exercise tolerance. The pain can radiate to the knee and anterior shin. Rest pain can occur and the sleep disturbed in more advanced disease. Patients complain of hip stiffness. Examination may reveal deformity usually flexion, adduction, and external rotation. Restriction of movement range due to capsular fibrosis is usual. Internal rotation is one of the first movements to be restricted.

Investigations

Plain X-rays may show the classic picture of reduction in joint space, sub-chondral sclerosis, cyst formation, and osteophytes.

Treatment

In the early stages of the disease, the management is conservative. This includes exercises to improve core stability, physiotherapy, analgesics, and anti-inflammatory tablets. Local warmth may be helpful. Lifestyle modifications and weight reduction may be necessary. An intra-articular steroid injection may serve as a holding procedure. This is usually performed under X-ray or ultrasound guidance. Visco-supplementation is another suggested procedure, although a firm evidence base is lacking. Arthroscopic debridement is also lacking a firm evidence base.

In more advanced disease, the treatment of choice is a total hip replacement (Fig. 9.17). This operation has been successful in improving the quality of life of millions of patients and is one of the most successful orthopedic operations performed

Fig. 9.18 Hybrid total hip replacement on the right side with an uncemented socket and cemented stem (Courtesy: Dipen Menon, Kettering, UK)

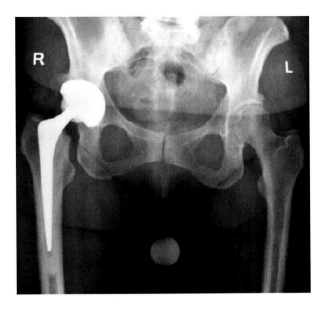

today. The operation involves the preparation of the acetabulum and the femoral neck to accept a socket (acetabular component) and stemmed head (femoral component), respectively (Fig. 9.18). The components can be cemented into place (primary stability) or rely on bone ingrowth onto the component's surface (uncemented hip replacement). Both techniques have their proponents. Hip replacements have a limited life span in the body (15–20 years) and it is best to perform this procedure in patients who are unlikely to outlive their artificial joint. This is however not possible in the young population with advanced hip disease. Performing joint replacements in this patient group is already increasing the revision burden and costs associated with this procedure.

Avascular Necrosis (AVN)

Avascular necrosis is a condition that results from damage to the blood supply to the femoral head. This results in repair and remodeling, followed by collapse of the femoral head and secondary osteoarthritis.

Causes

Post-traumatic: Following fractures of the femoral neck and dislocation of the hip

   Steroid induced
   Alcohol induced
   Related to pregnancy

Iatrogenic: Following treatment of congenital hip dislocation and slipped upper femoral epiphysis

Caisson disease: Deep sea divers and Tunnel workers
Idiopathic

Staging

The classification system used in most studies is the one described by Ficat and Arlet. This classification is based on X-ray appearances and is likely to be supplanted by more modern classifications based on MR scans.

Ficat and Arlet Classification

Stage 1	Hip pain with normal appearances on X-ray
Stage 2	Sclerosis of the femoral head with no collapse
Stage 3	Collapse of the femoral head
Stage 4	AVN with secondary osteoarthritis (i.e., acetabular changes) (Fig. 9.19)

Clinical Features

The condition can affect adults of all ages and both sexes. Patients present with pain in the hip which is usually constant and can be associated with a limp (Fig. 9.20). The pain is of insidious onset and can be severe, affecting the sleep and lasting for a variable period of 2–3 years. The changes of avascular necrosis can be present on an MR scan without any clinical symptoms or signs. AVN may be noted as an incidental finding in the opposite hip when a pelvic MR scan is obtained on clinical grounds for suspected unilateral avascular necrosis of the hip. The hip subsequently develops secondary osteoarthritis after a variable period of about 18 months to 3 years. The pattern of pain can change at this late stage from the constant pain of AVN to the activity-related pain of OA. The patient may walk with an antalgic or a Trendelenburg gait. Attempted movements can be painful and restricted particularly internal rotation in flexion.

Investigations

X-rays can help establish the diagnosis of AVN in stages 2, 3, and 4. A Technetium bone scan may reveal reduced isotope uptake in the avascular area and increased

Fig. 9.19 AVN in Sickle cell disease (Courtesy: Dilip Malhotra, Bahrain)

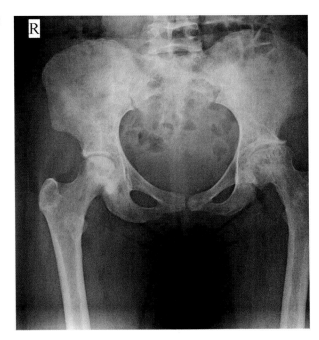

Fig. 9.20 Anteroposterior radiograph of the left hip joint showing avascular necrosis of the weight-bearing segment of the femoral head (Courtesy: Dilip Malhotra, Bahrain) (Reproduced with kind permission of Springer Verlag)

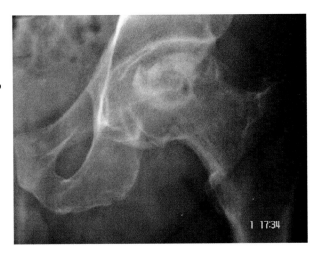

uptake around the avascular area representing the repair process. The MR scan is the investigation of choice to clinch the diagnosis (Fig. 9.21). It can also pick up early AVN even before the onset of symptoms.

Fig. 9.21 Pelvic MR scan showing bilateral avascular necrosis of the hip (Courtesy: Dipen Menon, Kettering, UK)

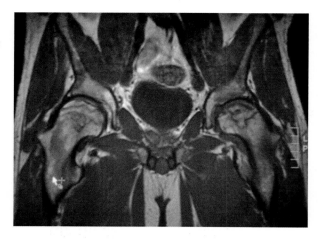

Treatment

In the early stages of AVN (stages 1 and 2), core decompression (removing a core of bone under X-ray control extending from the trochanteric to the affected area in the femoral head) can help relieve pain (Fig. 9.22). Core decompression does not halt progression of the disease process. Once collapse of the femoral head has occurred (stage 3), the available options are re-orientation osteotomies or a hemiarthroplasty. In stage 4 disease with intrusive symptoms, a total hip replacement is the treatment of choice.

Perthes' Disease

Perthes' disease occurs in childhood. It is characterized by avascular necrosis of the femoral capital epiphysis and associated remodeling of the femoral metaphysis and epiphysis. It occurs more commonly in boys than in girls. The blood supply to the femoral capital epiphysis is precarious in children at about the age of 4 years. The main blood supply to the femoral capital epiphysis at this age is from the lateral retinacular blood vessels. The postulated reason for the circulatory compromise to the femoral capital epiphysis is venous tamponade from recurrent effusions. Perthes' disease usually occurs between the ages of 4 and 11 years of age.

Clinical Features

The child presents with hip or knee pain and an associated limp. There may be a history of trauma though not in all patients. Attempted hip movements may be associated with pain and muscle spasm. Restriction of abduction and internal rotation in hip flexion is noted on examination.

Fig. 9.22 Coring in core decompression of the left hip (Courtesy: Dipen Menon, Kettering, UK)

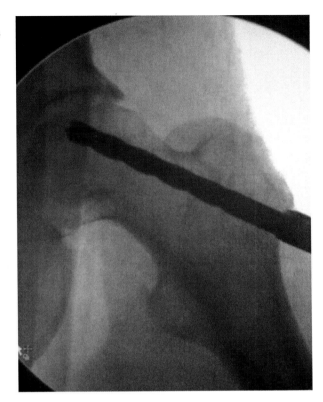

X-Rays

X-rays show sclerosis and fragmentation of the femoral capital epiphysis (Fig. 9.23). The greater the degree of involvement of the epiphysis, the poorer the final outcome. Preservation of the lateral pillar of the epiphysis is associated with a better prognosis. Serial X-rays show continued healing and remodeling of the epiphysis and metaphysis with eventual distortion in the shape of the femoral head and neck (Fig. 9.24). In severe disease, there maybe subluxation of the femoral head.

Treatment

The treatment of Perthes' disease is usually symptomatic (analgesia, intermittent traction, and physiotherapy) and continued observation during the stages of healing. Children under the age of 6 do well because of their remodeling potential with continued growth (Figs. 9.25 and 9.26). In some children, more aggressive methods may have to be adopted, particularly if there is evidence of hip subluxation on serial X-rays.

Fig. 9.23 Severe Perthes'
disease affecting all three
pillars of the right femoral
capital epiphysis (Courtesy:
Dipen Menon, Kettering,
UK)

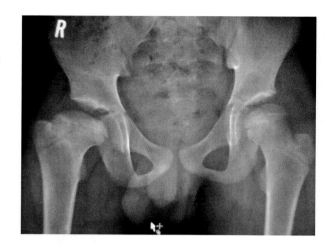

Fig. 9.24 Same patient as in
Fig. 9.23. Healing and
remodeling have resulted in
distortion in the size and
shape of the right hip
(Courtesy: Dipen Menon,
Kettering, UK)

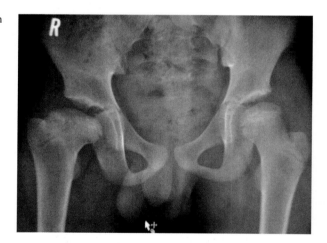

Fig. 9.25 Sequelae of
Perthes' disease (Courtesy:
Magdi E. Greiss,
Whitehaven, Cumbria, UK)

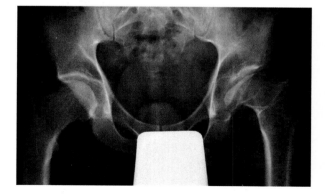

Fig. 9.26 Sequelae of Perthes' disease (Courtesy: Magdi E. Greiss, Whitehaven, Cumbria, UK)

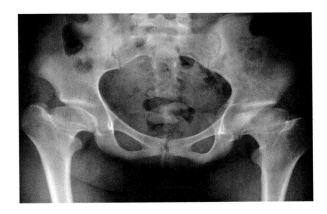

The hip can be examined under GA and an arthrogram performed to plan future management. Containment of the femoral head in the acetabulum can be achieved operatively by performing a femoral or pelvic osteotomy.

Chapter 10
The Knee Joint

K. Mohan Iyer

Anatomy of the Knee Joint

The knee joint is the largest joint in the body, and its integrity depends on its articular surfaces and also on the series of powerful ligaments and the muscles surrounding it.

The Quadriceps

The quadriceps extensor is made up of the rectus femoris and three vasti. It mainly extends the knee joint and is one of the most powerful extensors in the body. The vastus medialis is the most important component of this muscle since it is the first to waste following injury or disease and the last to recover.

The Popliteus

This muscle is mainly concerned with locking of the knee joint by producing lateral rotation of the femur over the tibia. It is in close proximity to the lateral meniscus in the lateral compartment of the knee joint.

K.M. Iyer
Consultant Orthopedic Surgeon, Bangalore University,
152, Kailash Apartments, 8th Main, Malleswaram 120/H-2K,
560 003 Bangalore, Karnataka, India
e-mail: kmiyer28@hotmail.com

K.M. Iyer (ed.), *Orthopedics of the Upper and Lower Limb*,
DOI 10.1007/978-1-4471-4447-2_10, © Springer-Verlag London 2013

The Medial and Lateral Ligaments

The medial ligament is a flattened band attached proximally to the femur and below and distally to the anteromedial aspect of the tibia. This ligament is in two parts, namely,

1. An anterior portion which consists of long fibers running between the femur and tibia and is readily separated from the medial meniscus
2. A posterior part, with short fibers and closely bound to the lateral meniscus, a little behind the midpoint on the periphery

Anatomically, this forms a mechanical weak spot where the mobile anterior portion joins the comparatively fixed portion of the cartilage.

The lateral ligament is a round band which stretches between the femur and the head of the fibula.

Behind the joint capsule is reinforced by a thickening known as the posterior ligament, which consists of an expansion of the semimembranosus tendon and forms the floor of the politeal space.

The Menisci

These are a crescentric portion of the fibro-cartilage which are arranged on the periphery of the upper articular cartilage of the tibia. On cross-section, they are wedge-shaped, with their thin portions being directed toward the center. Along the tibial spines the two cartilages form a hollow or depression for reception of the rounded femoral condyles.

1. *The medial semilunar cartilage*: This is larger and more oval than the lateral one. It is attached by two horns to the anterior and posterior parts of the non-articular surface of the upper tibia. The horns of the lateral meniscus lie within the embrace of the medial. Of tremendous importance is its relation of the medial ligament. Occasionally the anterior extremities of the two cartilages may be united by the transverse ligament.
2. *The lateral semilunar cartilage*: This is larger and more circular, with its horns attached to the tibia, and one on each side of the tibial spine. The posterior horn has a strong ligamentous attachment to the posterior cruciate ligament.

There is a well-defined groove on its posterior aspect just behind the midpoint, where the popliteus tendon passes across it.

Both the menisci play an important part in the function of the knee joint. They further the adaptation of the tibial socket to the femoral condyles, increase the stability of the knee joint, and also protect its articular surfaces.

The Cruciate Ligaments

The articular surfaces are also bound together by the two power crucial ligaments. The anterior cruciate is attached to the tibia immediately behind the anterior horn of the medial meniscus and passes upward, backward, and laterally to be attached to the posterior part of the lateral femoral condyle. The posterior ligament is attached to the tibia behind the posterior horn of the medial meniscus and passes upward, forward, and medially to the anterior part of the medial femoral condyle. The anterior cruciate is tense when the knee is extended and also when the femur is rotated medially on a fixed tibia. The posterior cruciate ligament is most tight in flexion.

The Tibial Spine

The spine consists of two tubercles, which are separated by an antero-posterior groove. The lateral tubercle is slightly smaller and some fibers form the anterior extremity of the lateral meniscus are inserted into it. The larger medial tubercle receives some fibers from the anterior cruciate ligament and occasionally the posterior horn of the lateral meniscus is attached to it. The size of the tubercles varies a lot, but there may be aplasia of the tubercles in some cases.

The Infrapatellar Pad

An intra-capsular and extra-synovial pad of fat is normally present just behind the ligamentum patellae. From its main mass, an extension passes backward between the layers of a triangular fold which passes posteriorly from the anterior part of the synovial membrane and the distal part of the joint. This synovial prolongation is known as ligamentum mucosum or patellar synovial fold and its edges as alar folds or ligaments. The fatty extension is called as the alar pad or the semilunar extension of the infrapatellar pad.

Integrity of the Knee Joint

Lateral motion of the knee joint in extension is controlled by the capsule, collateral ligaments, and the cruciate ligaments. In flexion, the same structures minus the fibular collateral ligament.

Rotary motion of the knee joint in extension is controlled by capsule, collateral ligaments, and the cruciate ligaments. In flexion, it is the same minus the fibular collateral ligament.

Fig. 10.1 Arthroscopy
showing chondromalacia
patellae (Courtesy: Dushyant
H. Thakkar, London, UK)
(Reproduced with kind
permission of Springer
Verlag)

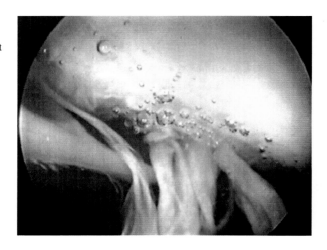

Forward gliding of the tibia on the femur is controlled by the anterior cruciate ligament.

Backward gliding of the tibia on the femur is controlled by the posterior cruciate ligament.

Lateral gliding of the tibia on the femur is controlled by the tibial intercondyloid eminence and the femoral condyles with the aid of all the ligaments.

Hyperextension is controlled by both collateral ligaments, both cruciate ligaments, both menisci, the posterior aspect of the articular capsule, the oblique popliteal ligament, and the architecture of the femoral condyles.

Hyperflexion is controlled by both cruciate ligaments, both menisci, the femoral attachment of the posterior aspect of the capsule, the femoral attachment of both heads of the gastrocnemius, and the bony structure of the femur and tibia.

The menisci cushion the hyperextension and hyperflexion. The tibial collateral ligament is closely related to the medial meniscus, but there is no strong fibrous-tissue attachment between them. The tibial collateral ligament glides forward and backward in extension and flexion.

Chondromalacia of the Patella

This is one of the commonest forms of degenerative changes in joints in the form of fissuring, flaking, or erosion of the joints. Osteoarthritis is a disease of the middle aged or older people, but chondromalacia occurs much earlier.

It is generally believed to start as a nodular swelling, more often in the medial facet than the lateral one. The articular cartilage loses its luster and it can be easily distinguished from the normal glistening cartilage. Fissures occur in a radial fashion with the articular cartilage in flakes (Fig. 10.1). The damaged cartilage is usually thinner and the bone becomes exposed and even eburnated. Osteophytes develop at the margins of the patella in later stages. Cyst formation may appear in degenerative cartilage. There are certain areas of cartilage cells that exhibit hyperplasia and the femoral condyles may show "mirror" lesions.

Some people also believe that traumatic subluxation of the patella with tearing of the medial capsule was a more common injury than realized. Such a recurrent phenomenon can cause chondromalacia patellae. The femoral surface of the patella is made up of seven articular facets for articulation with the femoral condyles, during flexion and extension, and it is the medial facet that is involved most.

Clinical Features

The patient is normally a young adult with a history of injury or a twist. Initially discomfort rather than pain is felt. The pain is felt immediately behind the patella and is marked during period of activity. Even osteoarthritis is an uncommon development. There is pain rubbing the patella on the femur along with tenderness on pressing the patella on the femoral condyles.

Radiographs are usually taken in the tangential view, and the irregularity is clearly seen.

Treatment

Medical therapy with rest and salicylates and quadriceps exercises is very helpful in most cases. Continued pain despite medical treatment indicates the need to consider operative treatment.

It has been well accepted that patellectomy is far more superior than other forms of operative treatment, such as shaving which is avoided when there large areas are involved.

Habitual or Recurrent Dislocation of the Patella

The patella may be displaced because of injury or a congenital abnormality.

It may be dislocated upward, medially, or laterally, though a lateral displacement is very rare. Medial dislocation usually results from injury or in severe forms of genu varum. Occasionally, as a result of injury, the bone may rotate along its longitudinal axis in such a way that one of its border is caught between the condyles of the femur, and even this is an extremely rare thing. The upward dislocation is usually traumatic in origin or in usually neglected rupture of the ligamentum patellae. The commonest type is the lateral variety which may become recurrent or habitual in course of time. Its causes can be as follows:

Fig. 10.2 Habitual
dislocation of the patella due
to congenital flattening of the
articular surface of the patella
(Courtesy: Magdi E. Greiss,
Whitehaven, Cumbria, UK)

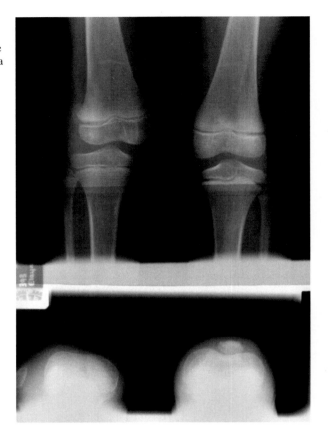

1. An abnormally high patella which is seen in an Osgood-Schlatter disease.
2. *Congenital causes*: Cases with poor development of the lateral femoral condyle, congenital anomalies of the patella (Fig. 10.2), malattachment of the iliotibial tract, and in external rotation of the tibia or the nail-patella syndrome.
3. *Rachitic causes*: Lateral displacement of the patella may occur with rachitic genu valgum. As the knee flexes in such cases, the patella usually slips over the lateral femoral condyle.
4. *Traumatic causes*: This type usually occurs in the adolescent female and is often associated with genu valgum or an extra long ligamentum patellae.

Clinical Features

Usually the patella slips out momentarily over the lateral femoral condyle and the patient complains of giving way with synovitis following this. Each recurrence is usually precipitated by sudden muscular contraction of the quadriceps when the knee is semi-flexed or flexed and the foot is everted so that the insertion of the ligamentum lies more laterally.

In recurrent or habitual dislocation, there is very little pain felt. It is only in the late stage when there is considerable pain, disability, or swelling of the joint.

The quadriceps and the vastus medialis is wasted and the patellar tendon usually lax. Lateral movement of the patella is more than the medial movement and radiographs may show the patella which is placed higher and laterally than it usually is.

Reduction is very easy. The knee is extended and then flexed to relax the quadriceps. The patella is then manipulated into its position by pushing it medially, at the same time correcting rotation.

Treatment

Conservative Treatment

This is of great importance when the condition is early, when the patient is instructed to walk with the toes inturned.

Operative Treatment

A wide choice of operations is available and the final decision depends on the cause of the condition.

1. *Osteotomy*: If knock-knee is the cause, then a supracondylar osteotomy is carried out with a pop cast for 6–8 weeks, followed by physiotherapy.
2. *Transplantation of the tibial tuberosity as described by Hauser*: The tibial tuberosity with a block of bone is transplanted anteromedially and this is then fixed by a compression screw. Post-operatively the knee is given a compression bandage for 3 weeks, when the sutures are removed and above knee POP cast is given. One has to be very cautious for growth disturbances and, hence for children above the age of 13 years, the patellar tendon is split longitudinally and its outer half detached from the tibia and passed behind the inner portion to be sutured into the osteo-periosteal tissues of the upper tibia as well as fascia overlying the Sartorius muscle.

Bursitis of the Knee

See Chapter 17 in my book entitled 'General principles of Orthopedics and Tauma' (Springer).

Flexion Contracture of the Knee

This condition is commonly a sequel to the continued over-action of the hamstring tendon. It is also seen in neglected tuberculosis and in rheumatoid arthritis. There are mainly two types of flexion contractures, namely,

1. A simple contracture in which a release of the tight posterior structures by division or stretching permitted the upper end of the tibia to glide around the femoral condyle into full extension.
2. In which even though a division of the contracted posterior structures, the upper end of the tibia, hinged at its anterior edge, instead of gliding around the femoral condyle subluxates posteriorly. This can be helped by division of the anterior cruciate ligament so that the subluxated tibia can ride forward.

Certain operative procedures can be helpful if conservative treatment fails.

1. *Posterior capsulotomy*: This procedure is best approached through two lateral incisions. The iliotibial band is divided transversely and the peroneal nerve isolated, and the biceps lengthened in a Z-manner. Through a medial incision above the adductor tubercle and with the knee in flexion, the capsular structures in the region of the intercondylar notch are freed, divided, or lengthened as per requirements. When the cortices are nearing an osteotomy, a manipulation is gently done to get a straight knee. Post-operatively an above knee POP cast is given for 3 weeks and later converted to a walking pop cast for 2 months.
2. *Osteotomy*: When there is free movement from 30° to 100°, a wedge osteotomy with its base anteriorly at the supracondylar level can be carried out. An internal fixation with a plate allows for early movement of the knee.

The Stiff Knee

The commonest factor in a problem knee is the presence of adhesions. These may occur within the synovial cavity, especially the suprapatellar pouch, in the capsular and peri-articular tissue, in the quadriceps, and in the fascia lata. Limitation of flexion at the knee is commonly found in fractures in the vicinity of the knee, particularly fracture of the shaft of the femur, after infections in and about the knee joint, and following certain operations where the knee is kept extended for long periods.

Most of these produce stiffness for obvious reasons. When a fracture is uniting slowly possibly because of treatment, the knee is very likely to be stiff thereafter. The prevention is to secure union as quickly as possible. In cases necessitating exposure of the shaft of the femur, the anatomical approach without dividing too much of muscles or dividing many vessels is important. It should be possible to go between the muscles, as for example that used in a posterolateral approach.

The complication following fracture of the femur may result from fragment entering the knee joint. Prolonged skeletal traction especially if the pin is through the lower end of the femur and especially if the knee is fixed for too long, such as 7–8 weeks, but almost certainly results in difficulty of knee movements.

Limitation of Movement of the Knee in Extension

This commonly results after fibrous ankylosis resulting from injury involving the quadriceps mechanism or the suprapatellar pouch, prolonged immobilization particularly for delayed union or non-union of a fractured femur or inflammation. It is of interest that the vastus intermedius is usually most affected by fibrosis and adhesion with the rectus femoris or vastus medialis being rarely involved.

Some workers have reported the results of operation by a straight midline incision, when the expansions of the vastus medialis and lateralis were detached from the patellar ligament and quadriceps from each side. Adhesions were divided to give full flexion. The results of this procedure were good.

Many workers have reported the results of quadricepsplasty with an average gain in the range of flexion till 70°. Full extension was gained in those cases where lengthening of the rectus femoris was not carried out. A progressive fibrosis of vastus intermedius was also seen by some workers.

Fibrotic contracture of the quadriceps muscle mass produces restriction of flexion, both active and passive, especially when the vastus intermedius is involved.

Considerable experience has shown that all parts of the quadriceps may be involved as well as the iliotibial tract, except the vastus medialis, for all these to require correction to obtain a reasonable range of flexion.

Treatment

1. *Manipulation*: Manipulation is contraindicated in the presence of a pathological process, indicated by a "hot spot" in the early stages of recovery, in the presence of any decalcification of the adjacent bones and in the presence of unsound union at the fracture site. If the patella is relatively mobile, there is no fibrosis in the suprapatellar region and the resistance is elastic with the manipulation being successful. Apart from the reaction and failure, a fracture of the patella is to be feared. Following manipulation, supervised active exercises are carried out persistently with vigor. An alternative in such cases and in cases where manipulation is contraindicated, some form of operation is considered.
2. *Quadricepsplasty*: The incision is on the lateral side of the thigh and it extends from above the patella to the upper thirds of the thigh. The rectus is isolated and separated from the vastus lateralis and the vastus medialis. The anterior knee

capsule is divided transversely on both sides of the patella for a significant distance to overcome the capsular shortening. The vastus intermedius which is finally scarred fixing the patella and the rectus femoris to the femur and obliterating the suprapatellar pouch is completely excised leaving the fibrous and periosteal covering on the anterior surface of the femur. The knee is then slowly flexed releasing the adhesions. If the vasti are badly scarred, then they are isolated from the rectus by suture of the subcutaneous tissue and fat to the anterior surface of the femur, thereby creating an artificial intermuscular septum and eliminating all scarred muscle from the remaining quadriceps. If the vasti are relatively normal, they are re-united to the rectus as far distally as the lower third of the thigh. After operation, the leg is placed in a Thomas' splint with skin traction to the knee for 4 weeks, after which active exercises are started immediately.

Injuries and Displacements of the Semilunar Cartilages

Mechanism of Displacement

1. *The Medial Semilunar Cartilage*:
   Normally the medial semilunar cartilage glides slightly backward when the knee is flexed. If the joint at the same time is abducted and the medial compartment of the knee is opened up, the mobility of the cartilage is still further increased. Sudden medial rotation of the femur on the fixed tibia forces the medial meniscus toward the back of the joint. The medial rotation causes the ligament to become taut, and the ligament at first steadies the posterior part of the cartilage. If the ligament withstands the strain, therefore the anterior movable part of the cartilage bears the brunt of the injury. It may either be detached from the junction with the fixed part or it may undergo any variety of the transverse or oblique tear. The fragment slips into the interior of the joint, and then when extension is attempted and an endeavor made to "screw the condyle home," the fragment is ripped or impacted between the condyles and the knee "locks."

   When the rotatory strain is severe, the medial ligament may be stretched that the connection between it and the cartilage is destroyed. The ligament may be detached from its tibial attachment and from the cartilage. In either event, the whole cartilage slips into the interior of the joint, and as extension of the knee occurs, the free border is between the condyles and a longitudinal slit occurs in the substance of the cartilage, when it is called as a "bucket handle tear." When such a tear involves the posterior third of the meniscus, it springs back into place and locking does not occur.
2. *The lateral semilunar cartilage*: The lateral semilunar cartilage is less frequently injured than the medial, since it is more mobile and is not attached to the lateral ligament. Nevertheless, severe degrees of violence may result in tears or displacements.

   The anterior horn may be torn if the femur is forcibly rotated outward on the fixed tibia, when the knee is flexed. Medial rotation of the femur on the fixed tibia combined with violent flexion is liable to cause a lesion of the posterior horn.

Injuries to either cartilages occur only when the knee joint is in flexion and the reason for this is because the cartilages are firmly fixed to the head of the tibia and thus follow it in all movements. If the knee joint is bent at the time of receiving the strain, then a lateral or rotatory strain on the joint may easily displace the cartilage from its attachment to the tibia.

Pathology of Semilunar Cartilage Injuries

The commonest injury of the medial meniscus is called the "bucket handle tear." It mainly consists of a longitudinal fracture through the substance of the meniscus, causing the fractured portion to be displaced into the center of the joint, with the anterior and posterior attachments remaining intact. Almost all remaining lesions of the menisci consist of some form of bucket handle tear with or without modifications caused by subsequent trauma, e.g., a longitudinal fracture may also occur through the substance of the anterior third in which event one limb usually retains its attachment and the other is mobile and slips into the joint cavity. A similar type of injury is found in association with the posterior horn injuries.

Further examples occur when the centrally displaced portion of a complete bucket handle tear is subjected to a further longitudinal split or is torn transversely leaving tags of cartilage projecting into the center of the joint from the anterior and posterior horns.

In many cases, the cartilage loses its peripheral attachment and slips into the joint with movement.

A simple classification [1] of injuries of different types is as follows:

1. Longitudinal tears

   Peripheral or detachment – 10 %
   Complete – 23 %
   Segmental – either anterior or posterior – 2 %

2. Horizontal tears with either anterior or middle or posterior – 48 %
3. Cystic degeneration – 12 %
4. Congenital anomalies – 5 %
5. Regenerative lesions

Clinical Features of Displaced or Torn Semilunar Cartilage

Predisposing factors:
Occupational factors: This has been documented in the anatomy of the knee joint.
Lesions of the menisci are more common in miners because they have to stoop and their knees are always flexed in a squatting position to empty the shovel over their shoulder.

Certain forms of sport are commonly associated with cartilage injuries, such as footballers, hockey, tennis, badminton, squash, and skiing, all games that produce a sudden twist at the knee.

Racial differences have been described in the anatomical configuration of the knee joint, such as the Bantu miners have a low incidence of meniscectomies or in the Japanese having a greater incidence of tears involving the lateral meniscus.

Certain pathological conditions predispose to cartilage disorders, such as long standing genu valgum and recurvatum having the attachment of the cartilage weakened, recurrent synovitis, leading to distension of the capsule being associated with relaxation of the ligaments, among them the medial ligament, when the cartilage acquires more mobility.

Symptoms

An accurate and detailed history is very important. The mechanism of the original injury, whether by external force or rotation, history of immediate incapacity, whether there was a click, snap, or a tear, and the history of locking, weakness, or giving way should be noticed in the history.

The pain is situated over the anterior end of the cartilage, and frequently over the inner border of the tibia, where the short posterior fibers of the medial ligament are usually attached. In posterior horn injuries, the pain is more marked over the posterior aspect of the joint.

In recurrent cases, the symptoms are less severe than those accompanying the original injury, with a common complaint that the joint gives way or lets the patient down. These occur while descending stairs or jumping from a height when the cause of a torn meniscus occurs. Locking often occurs and when repeated, the patient learns by then to unlock the knee himself.

In the injury of the lateral meniscus, the history is similar except that the knee is twisted in the opposite direction and the pain is on the lateral aspect of the joint. Locking is rare, while clicking is usually felt and even sometimes heard when the joint is unlocked. McMurray described two diagnostic points in its diagnosis: (1) it always occurs at the same angle of flexion of the joint and (2) the angle is always 10° short of full extension.

Examination

The knee is examined anteriorly and posteriorly, both in the upright and recumbent positions.

Palpation for tenderness and integrity of the cruciate ligaments and collateral ligaments is also tested.

Movements: The full range of flexion and extension is tested. Lateral movements are also tested.

X-rays: This is done in every case as a part of routine clinical examination.

Diagnosis: The accurate history of a twisting injury along with a feeling of giving way along with synovitis presents the diagnosis without difficulty.

There is no frank locking but a sensation of catch is clearly felt. When the joint is slightly flexed, with positive signs, the lesion is more toward the anterior end. At mid-flexion and beyond, the damage to the cartilage is not much, and there is a transitory weakness followed by synovitis.

Most importantly, the knee can be manipulated so that the injured part of the cartilage is nipped between the bones. McMurray's test is performed in obscure cases when the knee joint is fully flexed so that the heel is almost placed on the buttock [2]. Abduction of the leg and lateral rotation of the foot will bring to bear on the medial cartilage a strain similar to that which produces the ordinary lesion. With the foot and leg held in this relation to the thigh, the knee is slowly extended. If there is a lesion of the cartilage at any point, from the level of attachment of the tibial collateral ligament to the posterior horn a distinct click is produced when the femur passes over the site of injury as the cartilage is usually thickened or loose. The same procedure can be carried out with the foot medially rotated. The patient complains of a stab of pain when the click is heard. A common finding is with a horizontal tear when there is a grating sensation accompanied with pain and tenderness on the joint line posterior to the medial ligament.

Certain tears of the meniscus can be aided by asking the patient to perform certain tasks, such as squatting. With a definite tear of the meniscus, the patient cannot fully squat without discomfort and can often point directly to the source of discomfort. Local tenderness may be helpful, with the anterior tears being tender anteriorly and the posterior ones may exhibit posterior tenderness.

Some of the results of meniscectomy may be overlooked by a tear of the cruciate or medial collateral ligament. Osteochondritis dessicans may simulate a cartilage injury and radiological changes may clinch the diagnosis.

When a patient who had a meniscectomy complains of pain, though locking has been cured by the knee, the possibility of incomplete removal or a retained posterior segment should not be ruled out.

The X-ray film should eliminate any bony conditions, such as a fracture of the tibial spine, loose bodies, exostosis, osteoarthritis, myossitis ossificans, and an intra-articular fracture. An arthroscopy or an arthrogram may be useful in certain cases.

Differential Diagnosis

1. *Injury to the alar pad of fat*: In these cases, true locking may be absent, though full extension is painful. Tenderness can be elicited by pressing on the pad.
2. *Rupture of the medial ligament*: Stress X-rays done with the knee flexed are very helpful in some cases.

3. *Rupture of the cruciate ligaments*: When the anterior cruciate ligament is ruptured, the tibia can be displaced forward, when the knee is fully extended. In posterior cruciate ligament rupture, the tibia can be displaced backward on the femur with the knee flexed at a right angle.
4. *Fracture of the tibial spine*: This follows a severe violence and not a rotatory strain. Locking may be the presenting symptom, and radiographs are helpful in these cases.
5. *Loose bodies*: The locking produced by a loose body is usually momentary and radiographs are helpful in these cases.
6. *Exostosis*: An exostosis in the region of the knee may interfere with the action of the tendons to simulate locking. Radiographs are very helpful in these cases.
7. *Osteoarthritis*: The onset is usually gradual and pain and stiffness are marked in the morning. This is usually diagnosed on X-rays.
8. *Recurrent dislocation of the patella*: It is not usually diagnosed on radiographs and the history may not be typical. This condition should always be excluded in women suffering from internal derangement.

Treatment

Treatment of the Original Lesion

Certain brief conditions apply to all cases:

1. Reduction must be accurate.
2. It must be maintained until the torn cartilage has healed.
3. The damaged structures must be guarded from any strain or further injury for a long time.
4. During this period the nutrition of the joint structures and tone of the related muscles must be preserved.

   (a) *Reduction*: Reduction is always carried out as an emergency, at the earliest possible opportunity. An anesthetic may or may not be used.
   (b) *Retention*: No splint is necessary. Immobilization with a firm compression Jones' bandage should be enough and quadriceps exercises are begun every day.
   (c) *Prevention of strain*: Abduction and lateral rotation of the leg on the thigh should be avoided. The simplest way of doing this is giving the inner heel a raise of leather.
   (d) *After treatment*: Quadriceps volume, tone, and control should be maintained by continuous quadriceps exercises.

Prognosis

It must be noted that only the peripheral part of the meniscus is vascularized and there healing in a bucket handle tear is dependant a lot on where the bucket handle is either toward the center or toward the periphery of the meniscus.

Without operation, the prognosis is fair in people with sedentary occupation, while recurrence of symptoms can be expected in a majority of patients engaged in manual occupation or people who continue active sports.

Treatment of Recurrent Cases

Operation is the treatment of choice in the majority of cases with the history of true locking and synovitis, and this is undertaken as early as possible before the onset of arthritis changes.

Controversy still exists between removal of the complete cartilage versus resection of only the damaged part of the meniscus.

It is well known that after resection of the cartilage, a "new" cartilage of fibrous tissue regenerates from the synovial membrane. While posterior horn of the original meniscus is left in the joint, the anterior horn regenerates and an insecure junction is noted between both the parts.

Technique of Operation

Pre-operative Treatment

The patient is taught quadriceps exercises, such as raising and contraction of the extensor apparatus.

The Operation

A straight parapatellar incision over the anteromedial aspect of the joint is carried out in a limb with the tourniquet inflated. The knee is flexed at the end of the operating table and the surgeon sits on a table facing it. The incision is deepened in layers till the joint is opened. The affected meniscus is grasped with a kocker's forceps and inspected completely. Any tears that are found are meticulously dissected with a sharp knife. The entire knee joint is inspected thoroughly and washed out. The incision is closed with one suture starting at one end with the synovial membrane and on reaching the capsule in layers the suture is tied off. The rest of the wound is closed in layers and a post-operative compression bandage or Jones' bandage with wool and crepe is given.

Post-operative Treatment

The very next day the patient starts off with quadriceps exercises till the day the wound is inspected for removal of sutures. The patient is then allowed ambulatory support with exercises.

Prognosis

Most people reported good results following this procedure.

Incomplete removal with leaving behind of the posterior horn is often associated with recurrent synovitis. Removal of the posterior horn can easily be accomplished by a short vertical incision behind the medial collateral ligament, with the knee in flexion.

Clinical Features of Lateral Semilunar Cartilage Injuries

The lateral meniscus is less frequently injured than the medial meniscus, mainly due to increased mobility. Locking and effusion are less common. The history, signs, and symptoms of displacement and tears are less clearly defined.

The patient may complain of pain mainly on the lateral side of the knee, with a sensation of something slipping under the examining finger and on full extension of the knee, the patient may experience a loud click or snap or a jerk, when the knee jerks back into place – the so-called "trigger knee."

Discoid Lateral Cartilage

Normally the human knee possess a discoid or circular shape before absorption of the tissues which causes them to assume the semilunar shape.

Clinical Features

The characteristic sign of a discoid cartilage is the loud click which is felt or heard during flexion/extension of the knee. This may be appreciated at any point in the arc of movement of the joint. It is actually an exaggeration of the clicking, which is so commonly found in traumatic lesions of the normal lateral semilunar cartilages. In association with this, there is often an aching pain on the outer side of the joint and a feeling of giving way of the joint. Locking is very rare.

This condition usually gives a history of trauma, and it occurs in young adolescents before the age of 18.

If the click is bilateral, the suspicion is strengthened, but a radiological examination is necessary in such cases to rule out an exostosis. Very rarely is there a widening of the lateral space on an intercondylar notch view because of thickness of the cartilage.

Pathology

The cartilage is thicker than normal and roughly quadrilateral with rounded corners. Not infrequently the peripheral margin curves upward to be attached to the capsule in the vicinity of the lateral femoral condyle. At times there may be a hypertrophied pad of fat in the anterior part of the lateral compartment of the joint, probably derived from the alar fold.

Treatment of Lateral Semilunar Cartilage Injuries

Reduction is often followed by a similar manipulation as described for medial semi-lunar cartilages, and retention and preservation of muscular tone are done in a simi-lar manner.

Removal of the lateral cartilage is essentially similar to the removal of the medial cartilage. While removing, it must be remembered that the popliteus tendon lies between the meniscus and the capsule.

Recurrence of symptoms: Symptoms may recur for reasons exactly similar to the medial meniscus.

A posterior remnant may require removal if indicated, by an incision just poste-rior to the lateral ligament with the knee in flexion.

Cysts of the Semilunar Cartilages

Cystic swellings in relation to the semilunar cartilages are fairly common.

They may follow an injury and are very common with the lateral cartilage, though sometimes the medial meniscus also is affected.

Pathology: The cyst is of varying size, sometimes multiloculated and usually on the lateral side of the cartilage. In addition to the marginal cysts, the cartilage is often studded with smaller cysts. The larger cysts posses a fibrous wall which may or may not be lined by flattened cells, the origin of which is still obscure. The smaller cysts are similar in nature with a mucoid material similar to that found in ganglia.

Etiology

There are mainly two views concerning the genesis of cysts of the menisci, namely,

1. They are congenital anomalies of the nature of endothelial inclusions, which become cystic due to irritation and distention from trauma.
2. They are cystic or mucoid degenerations in fibrocartilage, and fibrous tissue resulting from trauma, but without any previous abnormality of the meniscus.

Clinical Features

In the majority of cases, there is a history of trauma, which may even be some years ago. A swelling is usually present on the outer side of the knee, which is tense in extension and fluctuating and varying in size from a hazel-nut to a small walnut. Pain is always constant and with a few patients giving a cartilage history.

Locking is very common and very occasionally a snap or jerk may be noted in some cases.

Treatment: The ideal treatment is a complete removal of the cartilage and its related cysts. Only removal of the cyst often gives rise to recurrences.

Affections of the Alar Pad

From the synovial membrane which covers the deep surface of the infrapatellar pad of fat, a triangular fold passes upward and backward to be attached to the apex of the anterior extremity of the intercondylar fossa. This fold is called as the infrapatellar synovial fold or ligamentum mucosum and its free margin is called the alar folds or ligamentum alaria. The pad of fat lies behind the patellar ligament and the part of it which is carried in between the synovial folds and is frequently the site of hypertrophy or lipoma arborescens.

When the knee joint is extended, the patella is drawn up by the contracting quadriceps and the infrapatellar pad of fat is similarly pulled up to avoid getting caught between the femur and the tibia. When an excess of fat has been deposited in the pad, or when the quadriceps has lost its tone, the pad may not be sufficiently pulled up and is hence liable to be nipped between the opposing surfaces. Repeated trauma of this nature is associated with hemorrhage into the pad with further thickening.

In older subjects, the infrapatellar pad may be hypertrophied in association with intra-arthritic changes, such as villous hypertrophy of the synovial membrane.

Symptoms

The condition is often confused with Hoffa's disease. It occurs in young people and with mild injuries. The knee is painful, but the pain is constantly situated behind the infrapatellar ligament when only one knee is used. The joint tends to be stiff and the patient may complain that it is weak and liable to recurrent attacks of swelling or synovitis.

True locking does not occur, but at intervals the joint may appear to give way or a stabbing pain may occur result in the arrest of the patient's activity.

The pad on examination is usually enlarged and the swellings are on either side of the ligamentum patellae, which are tender. This tenderness persists or rather is more pronounced when the joint is fully extended. The quadriceps muscles may show signs of atrophy. Radiographic examination is usually negative, but some calcium may be deposited in the hypertrophied fat and may appear as a radio density in the situation of the pad.

Treatment

1. *Conservative*: The simplest way of treatment is to raise the heel of the boot on the affected side, which prevents full extension followed by subsidence of the swelling and symptoms. These measures are always supplemented with quadriceps exercises.
2. *Operative*: When conservative methods fail, then the operative removal of the pad is considered and the pad is removed.

Bipartite Patella

The patella arises from a single center of ossification, though in many cases 2 or 3 centers of ossification may be present. These centers fuse together to form a single centre, but in certain cases may remain separate giving rise to the condition of bipartite patella. This condition may pass unnoticed, but is seen very accidentally when radiographs of the knee are taken, particularly following injury.

Radiological Appearance

The general contour of the patella is not altered, but the bone may be seen to consist of a larger fragment and one or two smaller fragments, and this fragment is usually seen in the upper and outer quadrant. The consistency of the smaller fragment is the same as the parent bone, consisting of a shell of bone surrounding normal cancellous bone. The fragment has a normal rounded outer semilunar margin, but the margin next to the main fragment is linear and is seen in the AP view as a straight line. There is usually a radiological interval between the two fragments, which is made up of cartilage. In many cases, the condition is bilateral and a similar condition may be seen in the sesamoid bone beneath the head of the first metatarsal.

Diagnosis

This condition must be differentiated from fractures of the patella, in whom there is a definite history of injury and the usual features of injury are present, but the important radiological points are as follows:
1. The margins of the bipartite are smooth and consist of cortical bone, while the margins of the fractured fragments have serrated edges and involve cancellous bone.
2. The position of the intervening gap is also significant. Fractures rarely occur in the upper and outer quadrant as this is usually the site of the congenital anomaly.
3. The congenital error is frequently bilateral.

Rupture of the Cruciate Ligaments

The functions of the anterior cruciate ligament are:

1. The control of the forward movement of the tibia
2. The control of lateral mobility
3. The control of rotation
4. The control of hyperextension and hyperflexion

In the first function, it is the sole agent, while in the last three functions, it acts along with others, and hence an isolated tear of the anterior cruciate is very rare.

The diagnosis is usually made from the history along with a tender knee. Clinically the tibia can be displaced forward when the knee is flexed, and in some cases the tibial spine may be avulsed when there is unnatural mobility. Nowadays arthroscopy has helped considerably in the diagnosis of an anterior cruciate rupture.

The Posterior Cruciate Ligament

Its main functions are as follows: It controls the backward movement of the tibia (Fig. 10.3).

The posterior cruciate is taut in flexion and hence violence usually displaces the tibia backward over the femur when the knee is flexed. The most common cause of this is fall on a flexed knee with the impact being taken on the upper tibia instead of the patella.

The ability to clinically displace the tibia backward in a flexed knee is known as the posterior drawer's sign. Clinically there is posterior sagging of the tibia, with the knees bent in flexion to be called as the passive posterior sign. An isolated rupture

Fig. 10.3 Clinical photograph showing sagging of the tibia posteriorly, indicative of a posterior cruciate tear (Courtesy: Dilip Malhotra, Bahrain) (Reproduced with kind permission of Springer Verlag)

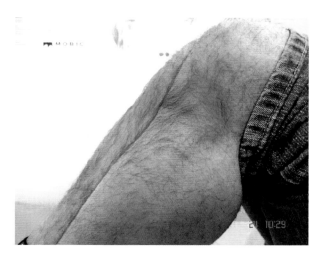

of this ligament is very rare and usually occurs in a severe dislocation of the knee often associated with other ligamentous damage and hemarthrosis.

Rupture of both the cruciates can accompany a dislocation when the knee joint is flail and the tibia can be moved forward and backward.

It is very important to note that a rupture of a cruciate ligament cannot occur without damage to other joint structures, particularly the capsule of the knee joint.

O'Donoghue [3] has contributed enormously on ligamentous injury of the knee. He has also shown how early repair of ligamentous injuries within the first 2 weeks gives good results in 55 % of cases, while late repair undertaken after 2 weeks following injury gives only 25 % of good results and reconstruction over 2 months gives only 20 % of worthwhile results.

Speed [4] has emphasized the following:

1. Tears of the meniscus with rupture of the anterior cruciate ligament, resulting in mild anteroposterior instability, but with no collateral ligamentous injury only require removal of the torn meniscus.
2. Tear of the meniscus, anterior cruciate ligament, and the medial collateral ligament requires repair of the medial collateral ligament.
3. The truly unstable knee requires reconstruction of the anterior cruciate and medial collateral ligaments.

Treatment

Primary treatment consists of aspiration of the hematoma through a wide bore needle and cautious immobilization to allow quadriceps exercises from the first day itself. Guarded immobilization should be carried on for the first 3 months, while the patient is ambulatory.

Treatment of Old Injuries of the Cruciate Ligaments

When the ligament has been ruptured for a long time, their ends become smooth and are covered by fibrous tissue. Considerable advance has been made in the diagnosis of ligamentous injuries by the introduction of the arthroscope. Even tremendous advance has been made by the arthroscopic repair of the anterior cruciate ligament and their evolution has been very rewarding as far as the results go.

1. *Recontruction of the Anterior Cruciate Ligament*: Whether this repair is indicated in isolated rupture of the anterior cruciate ligament or in association with other ligamentous injuries will depend on the individual given cases and the expertise of the operating surgeon. The most favored repair of the anterior cruciate ligament is by the patellar tendon or the semimembranosus tendon, preferably arthroscopically. The thing of paramount importance is maintaining the tone of the quadriceps in these repairs. This has been dealt with separately in relevant details in Chapter 19 in my book entitled: General principles of Orthopedics and Trauma. (Springer), on arthroscopy and arthroscopic repair of the knee.
2. *Recontruction of the posterior cruciate ligament*: Isolated tears of the posterior cruciate ligament are very rare and it usually is associated with other ligamentous injuries, such as the capsule of the joint. The efficacy of treatment as noted by O'Donoghue has already been described previously. Various procedures have been described for this injury which is beyond the scope of this book for a detailed description.

Rupture of the Medial and Lateral Ligaments

These ligaments are mainly involved in abducting and adducting injuries of the knee joint. The medial collateral ligament is more commonly involved. The lateral collateral ligament is often ruptured in association with damage to the lateral popliteal nerve either by stretching or complete rupture of the nerve. The diagnosis is made from the history, stress X-rays, or a diagnostic arthroscopy of the knee. The radiographs are usually negative.

Treatment

In an acute lesion, whether complicated with a nerve lesion or not, an exploration is justified and indicated. The ligament is sutured and the nerve is dealt with according to findings. Conservative treatment is carried out in incomplete lesions when an aspiration of the joint with immobilization is carried out. Care is especially taken when a medial collateral ligament tear is found as it is accompanied by a medial meniscus tear also. The medial meniscus tear is only diagnosed in later stages when symptoms arise.

Rotary Instability of the Knee

The importance of the instability was recognized in athletes running and changing directions while running. This may occasionally be seen as the end result of an unsatisfactory repair of ligamentous injury. It is usually caused by a medial capsular tear but may be accompanied by tears of the tibial collateral and the anterior cruciate ligament.

Clinical examination reveals excessive rotation of the tibia over the femur when the proximal tibia rotates forward and outward. Valgus laxity at 30° of flexion is present and is tender at the site of peripheral attachment of the meniscus and tears may be present as well.

At operation when the medial meniscus has been excised and there is excessive external rotation of the tibia, there is some underlying pathology. The operation is designed to convert this abnormal external rotation when the sartoris, gracilis, and semitendinosus muscles are converted to function from a flexor function to an internal rotator of the tibia.

Operation

The lower border of the pes anserinus is formed by the semitendinosus tendon, which is approximately 3″ below the base of the metaphyseal flare of the tibia. Using an anteromedial approach, the distal two-thirds of the pes anserinus is freed from the tibia with the knee at a right angle, and its lower border is folded up on to a point above the line drawn above the patellar insertion, but not above the medial flare of the upper tibia condyle. The flap so created is sewn under tension beginning distally to the periosteum and extension of the medial border of the patellar tendon. The muscle firmly supports the posterior condyle of the femur and tibia when this is done. Post-operatively a cylinder cast is given for 6 weeks, where after exercises are started along with weight-bearing mobilization.

Genu Valgum

This deformity is usually seen in rickets and may also be seen in the superimposed obesity with the femur being deflected to the lateral side.

This deformity may be due to (1) laxity of the ligaments, (2) quadriceps insufficiency, and (3) the child-bearing excessive weight.

Knock-knee is very common during infancy in children between the ages of 3 and 4 years when at this age children are found to have a knock-knee of 5 cm or more. Only 1–2 % of children aged 7 years or above have an equivalent amount of knock-knee. This is so common that it is often known as "idiopathic" and it is often caused by growth on the outer side of the epiphyseal plate at the distal femur. Here there is an inward projection of the knees and the leg deviates from the long axis of the femur at an abnormal outward angle. The deformity arises because the line of weight-bearing through the femur is though its outer side of the center of the knee joint. As the deformity is developing, the tibia rotates laterally on the femur, as a result of traction by the lateral hamstrings. Marked eversion and outward rotation are thus often present.

Usually a child of 4 years stands with the medial condyles of the femur and medial malleoli of the tibia approximately touching each other. Any marked separation of the malleoli, when the knees are in opposition, indicated genu valgum. When knock-knee is present, the child walks in an ugly manner since the knees rub each other and the line of gravity is transposed to the outer side of the knee joint. Falls are common and synovitis of the knee arises from joint strain. The deformity disappears when the knee is flexed since the posterior surfaces of the condyles with which the tibia articulates in full flexion are not affected.

If there is a deviation from the normal type of knock-knee, then an underlying cause must be looked for. Such cases are those where the knock-knee is excessive over 9 cm and where the deformity is symmetrical or where the deformity is in a child short of height for its age. This might be rarely seen in an epiphyseal dysplasia or in an endocrine disorder, or when there is family history of knock-knee or it could be due to a metabolic disorder, such as Fanconi's syndrome.

The progress is excellent if the amount of deformity is not excessive, over 5 cm. Correction usually occurs even if there is a deformity of 8 cm at the age of 3 years. This child should be under periodic observation and continued progress is an indication for active treatment.

Treatment

Knock-knee in children can be safely ignored and in children under 7 cm can also be safely left alone unless it is excessive and an underlying cause is found, such as rickets, or old fracture or renal rickets is found.

The only conservative treatment is to raise the inner heel in mild cases by 3–4 cm. This mainly satisfies the mother whose worry is thus helped.

In cases of severity, it is preferable to consider an osteotomy, with the osteotomy being carried out in the supracondylar region and mainly from the lateral side. Postoperatively the plaster is removed after 2 months, and the child given a walking caliper which is then supervised till the fracture unites.

Genu Varum

When a minor degree of tibia is curved anteriorly, it is called as anterior bow-leg. A minor degree of bowing is normal for a child up to the age of 3 years. An excessive amount of bowing is present when there is internal rotation of the legs along

Fig. 10.4 Clinical
photograph of bilateral genu
varum (Courtesy: Dilip
Malhotra, Bahrain)
(Reproduced with kind
permission of Springer
Verlag)

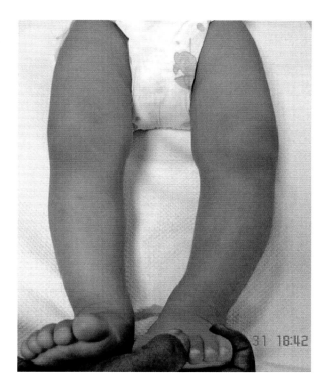

with obliquity of the tibial epiphysis. The bowing is usually restricted to the tibia, most commonly the lower two-thirds, there is always an inward rotation of the bone along the long axis of the femur (Fig. 10.4) since it is a flexible, three corned rod, and cannot be bent laterally without rotating. The toes are therefore turned inward when the child stands with his feet together and the knees are widely separated. On walking, there is a very conspicuous waddling that is present just like that of bilateral CDH.

It is very important to distinguish between the rachitic anterior bow leg and the saber-blade tibia of syphilis. In the syphilitic saber blade tibia, there is always some periosteal thickening along its anterior border, whereas in the anterior bow-leg, the thickening is endosteal on the concave side of the curve.

Childhood tibia vara can be divided into two groups, namely,

1. Those that are positional or dating back to intrauterine life
2. Those that develop secondarily to trauma or infection or to the peculiar form of growth interference called as Blount's disease

Bowing that develops secondarily to metabolic disturbance such as due to rickets or osteomalacia mainly occurs in the distal third of the tibia, and such deformities are rare.

1. *Physiologic bowing* (*postural, positional*): This indicates that the deformity will correct with further growth. This is true because part of the apparent bowing

Fig. 10.5 Blount's disease
(Courtesy: Magdi E. Greiss,
Whitehaven, Cumbria, UK)

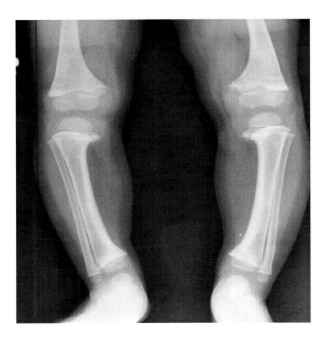

occurs through the knee on standing and stressing the knee toward the lateral side. This type of bowing is symmetrical bilaterally and it results in a medial facing of the distal tibia. The child must consequently pronate the foot to keep it flat when a chronic stretching of the medial ligaments of the foot occurs. Treatment is limited to arch supports by shoes or a pad, or both. Correction of future growth is usually seen in a child.

2. *Secondary tibia vara*: It usually presents between the ages of 1 and 3, with the condition often bilateral and symmetrical. The radiographs show a normal proximal tibial epiphyseal line and indeed the tibia often appears straight and bowing absent in a recumbent/supine radiograph.

Blount's disease is often unilateral or at least with a difference in severity of the deformity between the two tibiae. Beaking is prominent (Fig. 10.5) on the medial proximal metaphysis and is accompanied by fragmentation or irregular ossification in this area. During later development, the medial tibial epiphysis fails to gain in height and still later overgrowth of the medial femoral epiphysis is seen.

The underlying growth disturbance of the proximal tibia may well affect the result of corrective osteotomy. The end result may not be only of a persistent deformity but also a shortening of the tibia. Nevertheless, osteotomy is frequently indicated to prevent a secondary pressure on the cartilage and growth centers (Fig. 10.6) of the medial compartment of the knee between the ages of 4 and 7 years.

Bowing and tibia vara secondary to destruction of the epiphyseal line by trauma or infection brings a similar set of clinical considerations when the closure of the epiphyseal line may be necessary on the unaffected side to limit further deformity to obtain balanced leg lengths.

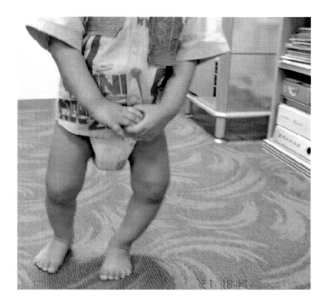

Fig. 10.6 Clinical photograph of Blount's disease in left knee (Courtesy: Dilip Malhotra, Bahrain) (Reproduced with kind permission of Springer Verlag)

Pellegrini-Stieda's Disease

In this condition, there is a characteristic presence of new bone in the region of the medial collateral ligament of the knee. A similar condition may also be seen in the elbows and ankles. The condition is usually seen in adult males and follows trauma along with traumatic synovitis of the knee followed by a period of improvement, although the knee never completely recovers. Movement of the knee is initially restricted and there is tenderness over the medial condyle, and the condyle appears to be hypertrophied on palpation. A radiograph reveals the lesion as a bony shadow beside the medial condyle which may be uniform or composed of a series of deposits. In the early stages, the bony shadow is hazy and ill-defined, but when the activity ceases, the lesion is clear-cut. They are usually first seen above the level of the knee joint in early cases, but are quite separate from the condyle.

Etiology

There is a postulation that the condition is just like traumatic myositis ossificans, wherein as a result of trauma there is a hyperemic decalcification of the medial condyle at the site of the attachment of the medial ligament. The development of ossification may be prevented by early recognition of the possibilities of the ligamentous strain that precedes the affection. An injection into that area with hydrocortisone, anesthetic, and hyaluronidase along with a compression bandage may be helpful in some cases. Passive movements are avoided as they can itself produce more bone and stiffness.

In established cases, a well marked area of calcification may not be expected to the full as the disease is self-limiting and as long as the case is not over-treated, a full recovery should not be expected in 2–6 months. Surgical removal is seldom indicated but might be necessary in some cases.

Loose Bodies

These loose bodies occur frequently in the knee joint. These also occur in almost every joint of the body and the main ones are mainly osteoarthritic loose bodies, synovial chondromatosis, and osteochondritis dissecans.

Classification of loose bodies

A. Fibrinous loose bodies (material of fibrinous material or necrotic synovial membrane)	
Traumatic	After hemorrhage
Pathological	In association with
	Tuberculosis
	Rheumatoid arthritis
B. Fibrinous loose bodies (composed of fibrous tissue)	
Traumatic	Organization of hemorrhage into villus
Pathological	With
	Tuberculosis
	Syphilis (gummata)
	Osteoarthritis
C. Cartilaginous loose bodies (Hyaline cartilage)	
Traumatic	Separation of whole or part of intra-articular fibro-cartilage
D. Osteo-cartilaginous loose bodies:	
Traumatic	Displacement of non-articulating epiphysis
Pathological	1. Detachment of part of articular surface, such as Osteochondritis dissecans
	2. Detachment of osteophytes, such as in
	Tabes dorsalis
	Osteoarthritis
	3. Separation of sequestra, such as in
	Tuberculosis
	Acute arthritis
	4. Synovial chondromata.
E. Miscellaneous loose bodies	1. Introduced foreign bodies
	2. Lipoma
	3. Angioma
	4. Secondary carcinoma, etc.

Fibrinous Loose Bodies or Necrotic Synovium

Typical loose bodies occur after a traumatic intra-articular hemorrhage and these are often laminated. Large numbers are usually present. The pathological type, namely those composed of necrotic synovial tissue, are usually associated with chronic synovitis or arthritis, particularly of tuberculous origin. They are multiple and form melon-seed bodies, which are very different from rheumatoid arthritis also.

Fibrous Loose Bodies

These may be attached to the synovial membrane or may be lying free in the joint cavity.

The traumatic type arises at the site of injury to the synovial membrane when there is usually a breach of the surface. As a result of this a pedunculated tag results, which sooner or later separates into the joint.

Cartilaginous Loose Bodies

These are rare and are derived from one or other semilunar articular cartilage.

Osteo-cartilaginous Loose Bodies

Traumatic Type

1. *Displaced non-articulating epiphysis*: This may be found in traumatic cases, such as in the elbow joint. This is mainly recognized by a limitation of joint movement. Radiographs are very helpful in these cases as it may be unrecognized at the time of injury because of a swollen joint.
   In acute cases, the joint is opened and the detached fragment is replaced to its position by a bone peg or screw or a K-wire.
   In late cases, the loose body is removed.
2. Detached portions of the articular cartilage – Osteochondritis dissecans
   This is a condition in which a fragment of the articular condition, with or without subchondral bone is detached either partially or completely, at characteristic places on the articular cartilage of certain joints.
   The joint most commonly affected and their sites are as follows: the medial condyle of the knee (Figs. 10.7, 10.8, and 10.9), but similar lesions are also found in the capitellum of the elbow joint, in the head of the talus at the ankle joint, and at

Fig. 10.7 Arthroscopy
showing an osteochondritis
dissecans lesion (Courtesy:
Dyshyant H. Thakkar,
London, UK) (Reproduced
with kind permission of
Springer Verlag)

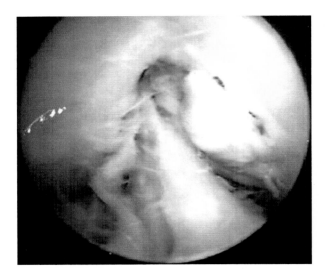

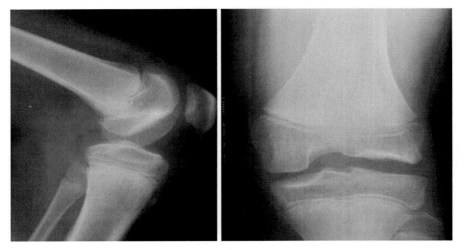

Fig. 10.8 Osteochondritis dissecans (Courtesy: Magdi E. Greiss, Whitehaven, Cumbria, UK)

the superior surface of the head of the femur in the hip, the head of the metatarsal. In many cases, it is bilateral in nature.

Smilie recognized three main types:

1. *Anomalies of ossification*: Because of the size and depth of the medial femoral condyle, alteration of the blood supply during periods of accelerated growth may be deranged if they do not heal spontaneously and this may lead to:
2. *Juvenile osteochondritis dissecans*: This occurs before the patient is of 15 years of age when accessory sites of ossification corresponds to this condition.
3. Adult osteochondritis dissecans.

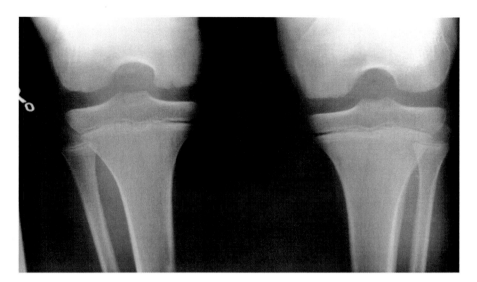

Fig. 10.9 Osteochondritis dissecans (Courtesy: Magdi E. Greiss, Whitehaven, Cumbria, UK)

Many alternative explanations are given for this condition, but the main theory is attributed to injury of the articular surface of the articular surface.

Pathology

The loose body may be lying free in the joint cavity or be attached to the articular surface by a fibrous band or by a hinge of articular surface.

Smilie also described other factors in association:

1. Instability because of meniscal tears, rupture of the anterior cruciate ligament, and recurrent dislocation of the patella.
2. Genu valgum with disturbance in the screw-home movement.
3. Decrease in the joint space by loss of meniscal tears or arthrosis.
   The appearance of the body varies considerably, such as it may be oval or with a plain and convex surface. The convex surface is generally rough and consists of cancellous bone, and this rough surface may be smooth when the body has existed in the cavity for a long time and the cartilage may proliferate to assume enormous proportions.

Symptoms and Signs

Clinically, cases have been placed in three groups, namely,

1. Here the knee is painful, swollen, and tender and locked in 15–40° of flexion. Radiographs may reveal one or two loose bodies in the joint cavity.

2. This group is mainly asymptomatic and it is found accidentally when X-rays of the knee are taken.
3. Here there is a definite history of trauma along with a chronically troublesome knee joint for 2 or 3 years, with a complaint of soreness and definite pain on weight-bearing and swelling. Some cases may have episodes of locking and the quadriceps is wasted in them. Very rarely can a depression be felt when the migratory body may be felt.

Radiography: Routine normal radiographs are usually taken in all cases in the AP, lateral, and condylar views. Tomograms are helpful in certain cases to outline the degrees of separation and may also help in localization of the lesion using a probe.

Treatment

The joint is explored when there are symptoms. The lesion is clearly indicated by a change of the color of the articular surface. If the lesion is movable, it should be scraped at its base and replaced to its base by Smilie's pins. If the cartilage is soft, sodden rough, it may be excised and all the loose bone removed, with the edges bevelled after excision. Smilie suggested that the loose fragment or about-to-be loose fragment should be replaced back to its original position and fixed with pins for removal at a later date when the fragment has united. The prognosis is good but the remote prognosis is less favorable because of the onset of osteoarthritic changes.

Pathological Osteo-cartilaginous Bodies

1. Detached osteophytes may be seen in

   (a) *Osteoarthritis*: Here three forms of loose bodies are seen such as synovial chondromata, detached marginal osteophyte, and detached "epi-articular echondrosis".
   (b) *Tabes dorsalis*: In the hypertrophic form of Charcot's disease, osteophyte formation may also give rise to loose bodies.
2. Two other types of loose bodies may be occasionally seen:

   (a) *Tuberculous sequestra*: These may be seen when large areas of necrosis like the articular surface of the hip when sequestra are usually wedge-shaped and are extruded into the joint cavity.
   (b) *Acute inflammatory sequestra*: This is occasionally seen in acute arthritis in children when a whole or part of the epiphysis may be detached and lie free in the joint.

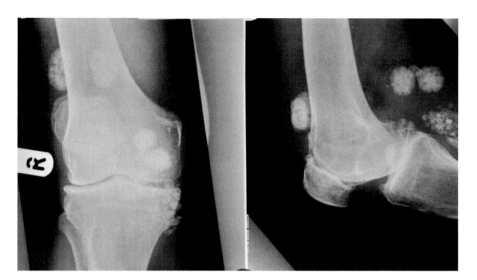

Fig. 10.10   Synovial chondromatosis (Courtesy: Magdi E. Greiss, Whitehaven, Cumbria, UK)

Synovial Chondromata

Many people believe that under the influence of abnormal stimuli, connective tissue cells may become transformed into any specialized mesodermal tissue of the body like bone or cartilage. Hence, synovial fringes may undergo cartilaginous transformation, which may later on become detached into the joint cavity.

Pathology

Such chondromata may be single or multiple and are occasionally diffuse.

The single chondromata which may be oval may be lying free or may be attached to the synovial membrane by a definite pedicle.

The multiple chondromata are smaller than the single type and are numerous in number.

Diffuse synovial chondromatosis is rare where the synovium is studded with numerous nodules (Fig. 10.10) and many undergo ossification and all have a central nucleus of true bone and many may be detached to lie free in the joint cavity.

Clinical Features of Loose Bodies in Joints

Usually there is sudden pain along with locking in a position of semi-flexion.

There may be an obvious swelling of the joint, and the loose body may be dislodged with a particular movement. In certain cases, an anesthetic may be required to unlock the joint.

After an attack, there may be an effusion along with recurrent synovitis and later on with lax ligaments and instability of the joint.

A notable characteristic point is the variable site of pain in contrast to cartilage lesion with a constant site of pain.

Atypical Symptoms

In the pathological type of loose body, the symptoms are masked by the major disease and hence the loose body is missed. Multiple loose bodies such as synovial chondromatosis are usually small to become more impacted frequently or may cause very little pain or inconvenience.

The classical traumatic type of loose body which is derived from the articular surface may be extremely difficult to diagnose.

Radiographic examination may be very helpful in the diagnosis of loose bodies, which are osseous or osteocartilaginous, when the radiographs may also show other co-existing changes. In the knee joint, an appearance simulating a loose body may be seen by a sesamoid bone in the lateral head of the gastrocnemius, which is always present in 15 % of all cases and frequently bilateral. It is normally recognized by its sharp-contoured oval or circular form in a constant position.

Treatment

Any symptomatic loose body should be removed. It is particularly very difficult in some cases when it is lying free in the joint cavity, when per-operative radiographs may be helpful in locating the location of the loose body. Or else a radiograph is taken with the leg in a wooden or radiolucent plastic splint when the radiographs are taken, which is removed when the patient is fully anesthetized in the operative theater.

Loose Bodies in the Posterior Compartments

When loose bodies are in the posterior compartment, the ideal exposure is obtained by a midline vertical exposure. Likewise for loose bodies in the posterolateral compartment, an incision parallel to the anterior border of the biceps may be used.

The lateral popliteal nerve lies posterior to the biceps and hence the biceps may be retracted backward and the iliotibial band is cut longitudinally and the capsule opened either above or below the tendon of the popliteus.

When loose bodies are located in the posteromedial compartment, an incision must be made along the anterior border of the Sartorius when the muscle is retracted backward and the capsule opened behind the posterior margin of the medial ligament, which opens up a small pocket that must be explored behind and distal to the posterior horn of the medial meniscus, where often the loose body is located.

References

1. Smilie IS. Injuries of the knee joint. 4th ed. Edinburgh: Livingstone; 1970.
2. O'Donoghue DH. An analysis of end results of surgical treatment of major injuries to the ligaments of the knee. J Bone Joint Surg Am. 1955;37A:1–13. 47.
3. Speed JC. Analysis of end results of surgical treatment of major injuries to the ligaments of the knee. J Bone Joint Surg Am. 1955;37A:1. 47.
4. McMurray TP. The semilunar cartilages. Br J Surg. 1942;29:407–14.

Chapter 11
The Leg

K. Mohan Iyer

Congenital Pseudoarthrosis of the Tibia

This condition is very rare. There is congenital abnormality of the bone in the lower half of the tibia (Fig. 11.1) and it is usually a pronounced anterior bowing of the tibia with a resultant fracture. This fracture is extremely resistant to treatment by the usual methods.

In this respect, this entity is unlike any childhood fracture, but the precise nature of the basic lesion which weakens the tibia is not yet understood. In some cases, it is often associated with neurofibromatosis. Every effort is made to heal this lesion, and unless it is done, the growth in the affected leg may be seriously impaired to such an extent that amputation may be the only answer.

Treatment

The best hope of achieving union is by an intramedullary nail along with cancellous bone grafting. This method succeeds if repeat operations requiring longer nails are carried out as the limb grows. Enhancement of the bone-forming capacity by the electromagnetic field around the tibia is worth a try.

In certain cases, the use of a vascularized bone graft increases the chances of success. The graft, such as from the opposite fibula, is transferred along with its arterial supply and draining veins which are anastomosed to host vessels by a microsurgical technique.

K.M. Iyer
Consultant Orthopedic Surgeon, Bangalore University, 152, Kailash Apartments,
8th Main, Malleswaram 120/H-2K,
560 003 Bangalore, Karnataka, India
e-mail: kmiyer28@hotmail.com

K.M. Iyer (ed.), *Orthopedics of the Upper and Lower Limb*,
DOI 10.1007/978-1-4471-4447-2_11, © Springer-Verlag London 2013

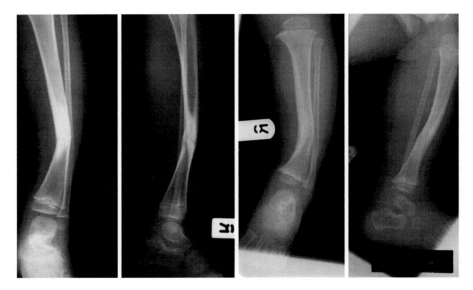

Fig. 11.1 Osteogenesis imperfecta with anterolateral bowing of the tibia (Courtesy: Magdi E. Greiss, Whitehaven, Cumbria, UK)

Another newer technique which gives promising results is that of bone transport based on the principle of bone lengthening by distraction of a growing epiphysis. By lengthening the proximal tibia, the whole upper fragment may be moved distally by closing the gap after excising the pseudarthrosis.

Another technique which deserves mention is the operation of threading an intramedullary nail after multiple osteotomies and this is conventionally called as the "sheek kebab" operation.

Osteochondritis Dissecans of the Ankle

This is a very rare condition that is often seen in males over 25 years of age. Initially they complain of an ankle sprain when they are missed and only 6 % of cases are diagnosed.

Ankle sprains are not infrequent and there is stiffness with pain. Clinically on examination there is a tender spot and sometimes there may be locking in case of a loose body.

A majority of the cases give a history of an inversion injury. In cases of a lateral lesion, there is a history of inversion along with dorsiflexion which shears against the fibula. In a medial lesion, there is a history of inversion with plantarflexion and impaction against the posterior tibial plafond.

Most workers agree with being sort of an avascular necrosis, though most agree with it being traumatic in origin.

In some cases, the osteochondral fragment may be disrupted in nature. When they are stable, new capillaries form and cross the fracture in an attempt to revascularize the fragment. If it is not stable or displaced, then it behaves just like avascular necrosis and fragments.

It is usually seen in 70 % of radiographs, even bone scan and CT are used, but MRI is the best in diagnosis.

It is treated in the following way:

1. In the early stages, it is usually treated in a non-operative way by rest in a plaster cast.
2. In the second stage, the same above treatment is continued for 6 weeks and 90 % of the results are good.
3. In stage 3, the medial lesions are treated in a non-operative way. The later lesion is treated by surgical intervention. In these acute lesions, an attempt to repair is expected whereas in the necrotic ones where the fragment is markedly fragmented, an excision is done along with drilling of its base.

If the condition is not responding to stages 1 and 2, then drilling is attempted to preserve the articular surface. This surgical intervention can also be done arthroscopically, except that in the lesion being medial in nature an osteotomy of the medial malleolus may also be required.

The results are about 88 % good to excellent in the long term and it is best if it is less than 1 year between injury and treatment.

In short, all ankle sprains that do not get better should be investigated. Doing an MRI is the best investigation. The lesion can be treated arthroscopically.

Rupture of the Peroneus Tertius

This is a very rare condition which has been described. This is a muscle located in the lateral compartment of the leg and takes origin from the lateral condyle of the tibia and head of the fibula, passes down behind the peroneus brevis, and passes beneath the peroneal tubercle to be inserted into the plantar surface of the first metatarsal and the medial cuneiform bone.

The patient complains of lateral ankle strain or hindfoot strain. On examination, there is tenderness on palpation along the course of the peroneal tendons. There is pain over the peroneal tendons just posterior to the fibula, and there is pain when the patient is asked to forcibly dorsiflex and evert the foot.

Rupture of the peroneus tertius is less commonly seen than a ruptured tendoachilis. Rupture of the peroneus tertius is also seen in rheumatoid arthritis, psoriasis, diabetic neuropathy, and local steroid injection.

There may be longitudinal slits in the tendon, and repetitive minor trauma may lead to attrition rupture of the tendon. It occasionally results in an incompetent superior peroneal retinaculum, which allows the peroneus brevis to rub against the fibula.

Basically there are three groups of clinical cases, namely,

1. Here there is no frank rupture
2. Here there is incomplete tears seen
3. Here there is a complete tear of the peroneus tertius tendon

The main complaint is pain. Initially conservation treatment is given a try before embarking on surgical treatment.

Chapter 12
The Foot and Ankle

K. Mohan Iyer

The human foot is greatly specialized in the following functions:

1. In standing, it provides for a stable support for the body weight, while its passive function is to provide for balance.
2. In walking, it provides for a lever by which the body can be propelled forward, namely, active function of propulsion.

It also functions in (1) conferring resiliency to the foot and (2) the arches function to disperse forces applied to the plantar aspect of the foot, in addition to the (3) passage of nerves and vessels forward toward the soles.

The Arches of the Foot

There are four main arches of the foot, namely,

1. *Longitudinal arch*: This extends from the calcaneus to the head of the first metatarsal, with its summit being the mid-tarsal joint. Certain variations in the arch may be achieved by alteration of the talonavicular joint.
2. *The transverse arch* is more evident when both the feet are placed together. This extends from the lateral border of one foot to the lateral border of the other foot. It has no true summit since the medial malleoli do not allow for complete apposition of the medial borders of the feet.
3. *The anterior metatarsal arch*: It extends from the first to the fifth metatarsal heads with its summit being the heads of the second and third metatarsals. This

K.M. Iyer
Consultant Orthopedic Surgeon, Bangalore University,
152, Kailash Apartments 8th Main, Malleswaram 120/H-2K,
560 003 Bangalore, Karnataka, India
e-mail: kmiyer28@hotmail.com

K.M. Iyer (ed.), *Orthopedics of the Upper and Lower Limb*,
DOI 10.1007/978-1-4471-4447-2_12, © Springer-Verlag London 2013

arch is supported by the transverse inter-metatarsal ligaments connecting the plantar aspect of the metatarsal heads.

4. *The internal arch* is formed by the medial border of the foot.

It is certain that the arches of the foot are present at birth, and on walking, the foot becomes flattened.

Mechanics and Movements of the Foot

The main movements of the foot are plantar flexion and dorsiflexion. When the whole foot is rotated internally about a longitudinal axis such that the sole faces medially, the foot is said to be inverted and the opposite movement is eversion. Both inversion and eversion movements occur mainly at the subtaloid joint. When the anterior part of the foot moves on the posterior part on a vertical axis, the foot is said to be adducted, while the opposite movement is called abduction. Both adduction and abduction movements occur at the talonavicular joint.

When the foot is in adduction and abduction, sometimes terms such as supination and pronation are used when supination consists of a combination of adduction and inversion and vice versa.

The normal neonatal foot can be dorsiflexed or extended by 45°, while plantar flexion is possible up to 50°. Likewise inversion and eversion are usually free without any prominence of the talonavicular joint or tightness of the heel cord.

Flat Foot (Pes Planus; Pes Valgus; Calcaneovalgus Foot)

Flat foot is either congenital or acquired because of an interplay of the following factors: (1) shape of the bony segments, (2) the plantar ligaments, and (3) the postural activity of the tibial group of muscles.

Clinically, there are two types of flat foot: (1) the calcaneovalgus foot, which is the commonest, and (2) the rare congenital type or the rigid flat foot.

The Calcaneovalgus Foot

This type of deformity is usually bilateral in 90 % with an inherited predisposition in 70 %, and its characteristics are as follows:

1. The feet are hyper-extended with the dorsum of the feet usually touching the shin.
2. The tendo achillis is not tight.

3. On plantar flexion, the anterior structures are usually contracted.
4. The talar head is usually palpable pointing downward and inward, which can be repositioned with reconstitution of the plantar arch.

This deformity is mainly treated by corrective casts with the initial position in equines and correction of the talonavicular and naviculocuneiform joints. This initial position is maintained and the equines is successively corrected for the first 4 months, where after the child wears arch supports till the age of 3–4 years.

The Vertical Talus Deformity

The characteristic features of this deformity are:

1. Valgus deformity of the hindfoot at the mid-tarsal joint, resulting in a dislocation of the talonavicular joint, and the calcaneus is tilted downward in plantar flexion rather than in valgus.
2. Correction of inversion is difficult.
3. The talar head is usually prominent and palpable, but cannot be manipulated easily back into its position.

Radiographically the talus is lying in a plantar flexed position with its head overlapping the antero-superior of the calcaneus, and after weight-bearing, the talus is in a vertical position, lying medial and anterior to the calcaneus. The talonavicular joint is dislocated and, in some cases, the navicular bone may be lying on top of the neck of the talus. It is interesting to note that despite all these changes the calcaneocuboid joint remains almost normal.

The etiology of this condition still remains unknown, and the soft tissue component plays a major part in its development.

Initial treatment by corrective casts usually fails, and surgical correction of the equinus deformity usually requires the need of lengthening of the extensor structures. This is usually done as a two-stage procedure, initially by capsulotomy of the talonavicular and calcaneocuboid joints along with lengthening of the extensor digitorum longus, extensor hallucis longus, and the cut tibial tendons to facilitate reduction of the deformity which is then held by a Kirschner wire along with an extraarticular bone block to the talonavicular joint that may be required in children of 3 years age or older. The second stage of this procedure involves a heel cord lengthening along with posterior capsulotomy and advancement of the tibialis posterior to the plantar surface of the navicular. This treatment is usually far from satisfactory and there is some chance of improvement when started early in the first few months of life.

The vertical talus deformity is also seen as a secondary "rocker-bottom" deformity following attempted treatment of a talipes equinovarus deformity.

Another type of a congenital flat foot may very rarely be seen in structural anomaly of the tarsus known as a talocalcaneus bridge or bar, which consists of a bridge of bone joining the posterior aspect of the sustentaculum tali to the outer surface of the talus. Any treatment is useless, and it is often diagnosed on X-rays. In very young children, resection of the bony bridge may help in relieving symptoms, although more often an arthrodesis of the subtaloid and mid-tarsal joints is usually carried out.

Acquired Flatfoot

There are various varieties of this variety of flat foot, namely,

1. *The osseous variety*: This variety may result from trauma to the bones or disease of the bones, such as navicular or calcaneus.
2. *The ligamentous variety*, which may follow rupture or avulsion from their attachments of the plantar ligaments.
3. *The paralytic and spastic varieties*, where the flattening of the arch is secondary and a late effect due to muscular imbalance.
4. *The static type of acquired flat foot*, which is the most common type of flat foot.

Etiology

The flat foot arises due to the postural muscles of the longitudinal arch being unable do their function when this arch transmits the body weight through a wide base of support.

Predisposing Factors

1. There is a general muscular weakness, such as is seen in convalescence after an illness. Severe trauma to the leg, which is complicated by muscular atrophy, is also a cause.
2. When the normal muscles are excessively fatigued. This may be occupational such as in nurses, policemen, soldiers, or following excessive exercise.

   Shoe wear: Unsuitable footwear can be a cause of many foot problems.

Pathology

In the early stages, the calcaneonavicular ligament yields, with the head of the talus being pressed forward, downward, and medially. The calcaneus is deviated to the medial side, with its anterior end depressed, resulting in a prominence on the medial aspect of the foot. The long and short plantar ligaments may also yield gradually, and finally the deltoid ligament of the ankle as well. When viewed from behind, the tendocalcaneus may appear to be deviated laterally along with overstretching of the tibial tendons and shortening of the peroneal tendons.

Symptoms

In the early stages, the feet are hot and burn after use, perspire more than normally, and the gait is clumsy and inelastic when walk everted and do not rise on the toes.

1. *Pain*: This is more severe on walking than on standing, because in standing the weak muscles relax and the entire body weight is borne by the weakened ligaments.
2. *Tenderness*: The commonest sites of tenderness is over the navicular, the inferior calcaneonavicular ligament and the sole of the foot, and frequently below the head of the first metatarsal.
3. *Swelling of the feet*: Localized puffiness is very common and, in some cases, edema of the feet may occur.
4. *Gait*: The gait is usually awkward and stiff without any spring. In these cases, raising of the heel is avoided mainly to prevent strain on the tarsal and metatarsal ligaments when the patient lifts the ball and heel of the foot together. The toes are usually turned outward, giving rise to "splayfoot."
5. *Pressure symptoms*: Usually the medial part of the sole of the foot wears out more quickly than the lateral side when the skin is more thickened and painful along the medial border, and painful corns may also be seen in weight-bearing areas, such as under the heads of the metatarsals. The lateral displacement of the foot may also rub the leather of the boot giving rise to callosities.

Types of Weak Feet

1. *Foot strain*: This is the earliest stage when pressure is exerted on the ligaments and there is no obvious deformity except pain and tenderness.
2. *Mobile flat foot*:
   (a) Due to faulty postural activity of muscles. Here there is a deflection of the body weight which disappears on standing.
   (b) Due to a short tendocalcaneus. The foot is in equinus, which disappears on tip-toeing.
   (c) Due to varus deformity of the forefoot.
   (d) Due to persistent fetal alignment of the femora, which results in abnormal internal rotation, with the patellae facing medially.
3. *Voluntary flat foot*: It is the stage where flattening of the arch has occurred with loss of postural tone in the tibial muscles.
4. *Rigid flat foot*: Here there are degenerative changes in the subtaloid joints.

Examination of the Foot

Inspection: Here the manner of standing and walking are noted. Deformity of the shoes is noted, such as excessive wearing away of the shoes or any bulging due to prominences.

With the patient standing, a line drawn from center of the patella passes through the space between the second and third toes, whereas in foot strain, this line passes to the inside of the great toe which is also seen when the foot is externally rotated on the leg.

The stability of the longitudinal arch can be restored by asking the patient to stand on his toes. The vertical line through the middle of the patella is again inspected, and when it passes medial to the great toe, the pes planus is of the rigid type and it is of the mobile type when it passes through the second toe.

It is also important to note the mobility of the subtaloid joint. When the heel is placed in the central or neutral position, the vertical line of the body weight passes through the second toe, and if this cannot be done, the deformity is of the subtaloid and mid-tarsal joints having lost their mobility indicating that the deformity is of the rigid type.

Palpation: This is done for any abnormal tender spots, indicative of a ligament strain, and pain is usually present over the sole in spring ligament strain.

Diagnosis

Certain conditions have to be differentiated, such as injury, arthritis, synovitis, bursitis, tendinitis, Kohler's disease, and osteochondritis of the calcaneus.

Treatment

General considerations: The main aims are:

1. To correct the abnormal center of gravity of the foot in such way that it passes through the outer side of the foot
2. To remove pressure symptoms

Treatment of incipient flat foot:

1. *Contrast foot-baths*: This may be beneficial in some cases.
2. *Electrical treatment*: When given to the small muscles of the foot, it increases their tone.
3. *Correction of footwear*: This is usually taken on a wooden model over which the shoe is built. In foot strain, it is important to thicken the medial part of the shoe so that it deflects weight to the lateral side of the tarsus and hence spares the longitudinal arch to some extent.

4. *Exercises*:

   (a) *Instruction in walking*: The heel-and-toe walk helps in building muscles.
   (b) *Exercises, active and against resistance*: This mainly helps in building up muscles to stretch shortened structures or strengthen relaxed structures.

   Additional exercises that are helpful are as follows:

   Tiptoe exercises
   Rising on the lateral borders of the feet
   Walking on the lateral borders of the feet
   Walking backward and forward on a supination board

   Treatment of voluntary flat foot: Here the deformity is mainly corrected by felt supports and spring rubber supports.

   Treatment of rigid and permanent types: Operative treatment is useful when arthritic symptoms have developed and when manipulation does not relieve the symptoms.

1. Talonavicular arthrodesis
2. Navicular-cuneiform arthrodesis
3. Extraarticular talonavicular arthrodesis

Peroneal or Spasmodic Flat Foot

This type may be seen in young adolescents when there is pain and tenderness with spasm of the peroneal muscles along with an eversion deformity of the foot. It may be of the following types:

1. *Congenital*: Certain anomalies such as tarsal bridges or bars or certain tarsal anomalies, such as abnormalities of the navicular bone.
2. *Acquired*: Seen in tuberculous lesions, rheumatoid arthritis, osteoarthritis, non-specific tarsal joint synovitis, trauma, and occupational strains.

   It is very important to differentiate between rigid flat foot and spastic flat foot. When the bar between the calcaneonavicular bone (Fig. 12.1) is complete, it forms a syndesmosis (cartilage) or synchondrosis (cartilage), and ossification may be there to form a synostosis of bone. This may result in degenerative changes in the talonavicular joint resulting in pain and spasm of the peroneals.

Treatment

This may be divided into two types, those with talonavicular bar and those with early rheumatoid arthritis or inflammation of the small foot joints.

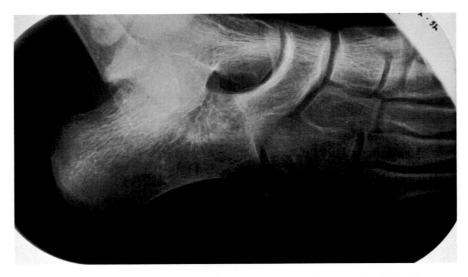

Fig. 12.1 Calcaneonavicular bar (Courtesy: Magdi E. Greiss, Whitehaven, Cumbria, UK)

In some cases, a manipulation under anesthesia followed by immobilization in a plaster cast may be sufficient for 6 weeks. Excision of the calcaneonavicular bar around 9 years of age may give good results. A subtalar arthrodesis or triple arthrodesis may be useful in certain refractory cases.

Painful Conditions of the Heel

Painful conditions can be classified as follows:

1. Traumatic disturbances
2. Pathological disturbances

Traumatic Disturbances

Effect of trauma: Pain is usually situated at the insertion of the tendocalcaneus or on the plantar surface of the heel.

When situated in the region of the tendocalcaneus, the underlying conditions are:

1. Tenosynovitis of the tendon sheath
2. Irritant bursae
3. Partial tears of the tendon

In all these cases, the pain is made worse by movements and is completely relieved by rest. In tenosynovitis of the tendocalcaneus, there is usually a swelling with an effusion, which is often accompanied by a fine crepitus, and when the condition is chronic, there may be an actual deposit of fibrous tissue in and around the tendon. When this fibrous tissue projects backward, the wearing of a shoe causes discomfort and this condition may also be known as "winter heel."

Bursal Enlargements

This may affect the bursa beneath the tendocalcaneus or also the subcutaneous bursa which develops over the most prominent part posterior surface of the bone. It is in the same location as an adventitious bursa forms due to friction of the shoe rubbing against the back of the heel. This bursa is liable to inflammation from friction due to an ill-fitting shoe, and hence there is localized tenderness at the site of the bursa and occasionally a small area of fluctuation may be detected by lateral palpation, anterior to the tendocalcaneus.

When the adventitious bursa is enlarged, the swelling is situated further down and is usually larger. Fluctuation is easily detected and the skin overlying the swelling is often red and edematous.

Partial Tears of the Tendon

This may result from forcible contraction of the tendon when avulsion of a few tendinous fibers attached to bone may occur or there may be a rupture of the tendon just above its insertion. In the first case, the disturbance of the periosteum results in a periostitis with minimal or no swelling, but tenderness exists at the point of insertion of the tendon. Partial rupture of the tendon may be associated in the acute phase with slight swelling due to effusion of the blood and later with the formation of irregular masses of fibrous tissue in the tendon.

Treatment

In all these cases, rest is a must.

In partial ruptures, when the pain is not severe, a heel raise from 1 to 2 cm may suffice to prevent over stretching of the tendon. In cases where there is a definite history of rupture due to injury, an early suture can be carried out.

In acute bursitis, rest is by rest from movement and, in subacute cases, the heel is raised by a sponge-rubber heel inside. In cases where the bursa does not resolve with this treatment, surgical excision of the bursa may be carried out along with the prominent bone.

Pain on the plantar aspect of the heel may be due to the formation of a calcaneum spur or due to an inflammatory fibrositis without any spur formation.

1. *Plantar fasciculitis*: Pain may arise at the insertion of the plantar fascia due to association with metabolic disease such as Gout or Rheumatism.

2. *Calcaneum spurs*: These are bony projection from the anterior edge of the calcaneum tuberosities, usually the medial which is also known as a calcaneum spur.
It is a sequel to repeated trauma or repeated attacks of plantar fascitis or due to
the constant pull of the attachment of the shortened plantar fascia or due to ill-
fitting shoe wear or it may be produced in the same way like a spur due to
hyperemia.

Clinical Features

When the calcaneal spur is due to a fibrositis or traumatic detachments of the plantar
fascia, the symptoms are minimal or none for any treatment.

The characteristic features are pain in the ball of the heel, mainly on prolonged
walking or standing, tenderness at the plantar aspect of the heel and most marked at
the attachment of the plantar fascia to the medial tubercle of the calcaneus.
Radiographs confirm the presence of a spur (Fig. 12.2).

Treatment

Non-operative: When the pain is acute, then rest is a must. Once the pain and tenderness have disappeared, proper shoes are given with sponge-rubber pads inserted
to relieve weight-bearing areas of pain. A rubber heel should be substituted for the
heel of the shoe with a cut just below the tender area.

Heat or short wave diathermy along with injections of hydrocortisone into the
tender area may be helpful in many cases.

Operative treatment should be reserved for the refractory cases and the spur is
removed through a medial incision.

Traumatic Subtaloid Arthritis

Fractures of the heel may occur by a fall from a height and they may not result in a
gross deformity, and only X-rays may reveal the fracture. Undetected fractures may
give rise to pain and weakness due a chronic subtaloid arthritis. It is best treated by
fusion of the joint.

Painful Heel due to Pathological Disturbances

Other than trauma, organic disease of bone or epiphysis and infection which may be
tuberculous, syphilitic, or pyogenic or may follow gonococcal or rheumatic toxemia.
Even Paget's disease must be ruled out.

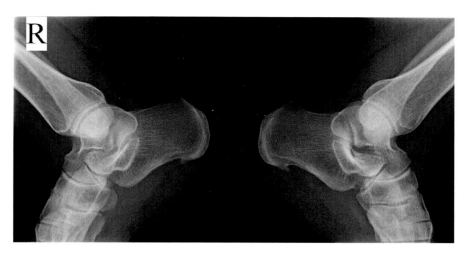

Fig. 12.2 Calcaneal spur (Courtesy: Dilip Malhotra, Bahrain)

Epiphysitis of the Calcaneus (Sever's Disease)

This condition usually affects boys in the ages of 9–13. Its differential diagnosis is as follows:

1. *Calcaneal bursitis*: Here the inflammation is more superficial and the radiographs are negative.
2. *Teno-synovitis of the tendocalcaneus*: Here pain is referred to the tendon along with a palpable silky crepitus felt. Radiographs are negative.
3. Bursitis between the calcaneal tendon and the skin, which is a superficial inflammation, usually the result of friction from a shoe and is readily recognized.
4. *Calcaneal spurs*: These are rare in early adolescence and usually found at the inferomedial aspect of the calcaneus. The tender area suggests the diagnosis and X-rays confirm the diagnosis.

Fibromatosis of the Plantar Fascia

Fibromatosis of the plantar fascia may result in nodules which are large enough to cause pain. It is very similar to Dupuytren's contracture in the hand and is relatively common in patients who take anti-epileptic drugs such as barbiturates and epanutin.

The individual nodules can be ignored when painless and removed when giving pain. Histopathology suggests a sarcomatous lesion with large active fibroblastic cells. Avoid placing a skin incision high on the medial side of the foot for fear of losing vascularity of the skin flaps. Excision is done by a lazy "S" incision, which traverses the medial half of the plantar surface to avoid weight-bearing areas that are subject to pressure from the overlying bone, but exposure is definitely on the medial side of the foot rather than along the side.

The Cavus Foot (The Claw Foot)

This is a condition in which the clawing of toes is combined with a raising of the long arch of the foot, which may either be congenital or acquired.

Etiology

1. *Congenital* such as spina bifida or a myelodysplasia of the cord.
2. *Idiopathic*, which forms the largest group.
3. *Acquired*: This may be subdivided into three groups, namely,

   (a) *Claw foot in infantile paralysis*: Claw foot may occur after poliomyelitis when the paresis is almost negligible.
   (b) *Claw foot in progressive lesions of the central nervous system*: This is a clinical accompaniment of Friedreich's ataxia, peroneal type of muscular atrophy, and other rare affections of the CNS.
   (c) *Claw foot following inflammatory infections*: It may be seen as a sequel to inflammatory contracture of the soft tissues of the sole of the foot.

Some believe it to be a weakness of the short muscles of the big toe as well as the interossei. Some believe it to be a weakness of the extensor digitorum longus with weakness of the tibialis anterior or it may be an overaction of the intrinsic mechanism due to a shortened tendocalcaneus or a loss of synergistic muscle control without any specific weaknesses due to the effect of poliomyelitis on the spinal cord.

Careful examination of the CNS must be made for wasting of musculature, any ataxia, or any muscle-power weakness, particularly of the long muscles of the foot such as the gastrocnemius or Soleus group. The ability to walk on one's heel and the reflexes should be tested. X-rays of the lumbar spine must be taken to rule out any spina bifida deformity. Bladder symptoms such as enuresis when present may suggest a CNS lesion.

Development of the Deformity

The intrinsic musculature normally flex the metatarsophalangeal joints and extend the interphalangeal joints. When the long flexor contracts on this straight digit, it slings up the head of the metatarsals and prevents a drop of the forefoot on the hindfoot. In the absence of the lumbricals, the long flexor pulls up the toes into flexion and no longer supports the metatarsal heads. The forefoot drops and the lax structures in the sole contract or "take up the slack," with the formation of a typical claw foot. The hindfoot in this deformity is normal, the condition being a dropping of the forefoot on the hind-foot, followed by a contracture of the plantar fascia and a clawing of the toes.

There is, in addition to the pes cavus, some adduction of the forefoot from the beginning. An element of adduction and inversion appears in the late stage of the process, as well as some secondary contracture of the tendocalcaneus.

Clinical Features

First-Degree Claw Foot

In this stage, the child is clumsy with frequent falls without any apparent cause. This was formerly attributed to a contracture of the tendocalcaneus, but it has shown that there is slight extensor weakness, with inability to pull up the toes.

Second-Degree Claw Foot

In addition to the slight flexion deformity of the forefoot, there is dorsiflexion of the great toe at the metatarsophalangeal joint and flexion at the interphalangeal joint. The plantar fascia is tense and contracted. The most important characteristic aspect of the deformity at this stage is that the deformity can be made to disappear by upward pressure on the ball of the great toe, thus showing that it is caused by a downward dropping of the metatarsal head.

Third-Degree Claw Foot

Here the arch of the foot is markedly raised and all the toes are fixed in flexion with the tendocalcaneus which begins to appear contracted. The plantar structures are fur-ther shortened and all the toes are dorsiflexed at the metatarsophalangeal joints and flexed at the interphalangeal joints. These deformities are fixed and it is not possible to correct them by finger pressure under the first metatarsal head. The main complaint is painful corns which develop at the dorsum of the flexed interphalangeal joints.

Fourth-Degree Claw Foot

Here, in addition to the cavus and hammered toes, there is adduction at the tarso-metatarsal joint giving rise to a kind of varus deformity. The foot is rigid and painful and there are tender callosities on the outer side and under the metatarsal heads, and walking becomes very painful and difficult.

Fifth-Degree Claw Foot

This is usually seen in cases following some paralytic condition when the toes become blue and cold and the whole foot is contracted into a rigid equinovarus with a high arch. The patient is extremely disabled with markedly tender callosities.

Treatment

First Degree

The progress is arrested by re-educating small muscle function and by exercises that strengthen the foot in general. Shoes are mainly fitted with a 1 cm thick metatarsal bar placed across the sole of the foot, immediately behind the heads of the metatarsal bones. Shoes without any heels are helpful.

Second Degree

A shoe is fitted to give some temporary relief till the definitive operation, which consists of subcutaneously dividing the plantar fascia and the tendon of the extensor proprius hallcis is divided at its insertion and passed through the neck of the first metatarsal. Arthrodesis of the interphalangeal joint is done in a straight plane which improves the take-off phase of gait. A POP cast is then applied to the foot to maintain it in a corrected position, which is taken off after 4 weeks and a metatarsal bar then given to the shoe.

Third Degree

Treatment is more of a necessity than in the second stage, though more extensive in nature.

All the structures arising from the calcaneus are separated from the bone forward and hence this procedure is a muscle-slide operation. The extensor tendons of the toes which may lead to relapse are then divided. A horizontal osteotomy of the calcaneus with a slide forward of the lower half is very helpful in some cases.

Lambrinudi's Operation

The main principle is that by arthrodesis of the interphalangeal joints, the long flexor muscles take up the function of the lumbricals and flex the toes at the metatarsophalangeal joints, and themselves sling up the metatarsal heads tending to straighten out the foot. This operation causes considerable improvement of the deformity, with reduction of symptoms from corns and callosities, and also a marked improvement in the general function of the foot.

Girdlestone Tendon Transfer Operation

The long and short toe flexors are brought out through the lateral aspect of the proximal phalanyx and then sutured onto the extensor expansion. A dorsal capsulotomy of the metatarsophalangeal joint may be necessary in some cases. A cast may be applied for 6 weeks. This operation is particularly indicated and helpful in the young individual with marked soft-tissue contractures.

Fourth and Fifth Degrees

In the fourth stage, the high crooked arch can be corrected only by dividing the bones across at the level of the mid-tarsal joint. If the deformity is very rigid, then a triple arthrodesis of Naughton-Dunn may be considered.

Congenital Talipes Equinovarus (Club Foot)

This is a deformity in which the foot is turned inward to a varying degree.

Classically there are four elements to this deformity, namely, (1) flexion of the ankle, (2) inversion of the foot, (3) adduction of the forefoot, and (4) medial rotation of the tibia.

Etiology

Club foot may result from an osseous, muscular, or neuropathic error when it is termed as idiopathic.

Environmental factors such as intrauterine compression by a change in the size of the uterus or reduction in the amount of amniotic fluid have been postulated over many years.

Certain anatomic disturbances as seen in the talocalcaneal joint, in the innervation of the peroneal muscles, and in the insertion of the tibialis posterior have been described.

Genetic factors or polygenetic factors in the form of an autosomal-dominant inheritance with reduced penetrance were present in a small family group.

There are mainly two types that are recognized: (1) majority which respond well to conservative treatment and (2) a minority which are resistant to correction even by operation.

Pathological Anatomy

The typical club foot is at first a deformity of the soft tissue only. The essential features are plantar flexion of the talus, inversion of the calcaneus, and adduction of the forefoot.

Basically at birth the bones are normal in shape but altered in position. There are mainly three degrees of error which may be distinguished. In the first one, there is only forefoot error, in the second one inversion and equinus are present along with adduction, and in the third degree, the toes are pointing directly upward and the sole may be in contact with the medial surface of the tibia, and there is inversion and adduction of the forefoot but no equinus deformity.

Muscle and Tendon

The muscles are poorly developed and the tendons delicate. The tendocalcaneus passes downward and inward to its insertion into the calcaneus while the plantar muscles, especially on the medial side, are contracted and the anterior muscles of the leg are elongated (Fig. 12.3).

The Ligaments

The ligaments on the medial and lateral surfaces of the talocalcananeonavicular joints are contracted and the plantar calcaneonavicular ligament being very small, with the deltoid ligament of the ankle similarly affected.

Bones

1. *The talus*: The head and neck of the talus are deflected downward and medially, carrying with it the navicular and forefoot.
2. *The calcaneus*: The calcaneus becomes tilted so that its medial tuberosity approaches the medial malleolus.
3. *The navicular and the cuboid*: They are displaced inward and the toes are plantarflexed.

   In addition to all the above changes, it is assumed that the tibia is rotated medially.

Clinical Features

In a small proportion of cases, the structural bony changes are present at birth, and this type is distinguished by the presence of a small inverted heel and hard shrunken

Fig. 12.3 Clinical photograph showing bilateral club feet (Courtesy: Dilip Malhotra, Bahrain) (Reproduced with kind permission of Springer and Verlag)

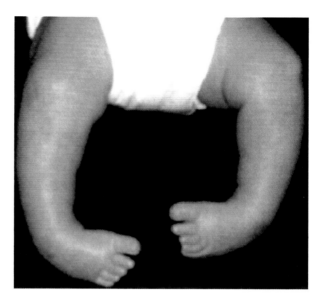

calf muscles, the condition itself suggesting a primary myelodysplasia. It is this type that is difficult to treat and maintain.

In unilateral cases, the deformity is never as severe but the leg is obviously smaller and less developed as compared to the other side.

The skin may be normal and stretched and thin on the dorsum, and thrown into creases on the medial border and the sole.

The head of the talus may be felt on the dorsum of the foot, while the lateral border of the foot may be convex and the medial border concave. The forefoot is plantarflexed on the hindfoot, with the heel rotated medially and upward throwing the whole foot into equinus. In many cases, a genu valgum may be present.

Diagnosis

The diagnosis is easy, but it must be remembered that an inverted position is frequently assumed in young infants. It can be over-corrected by gentle manipulation and the foot can be dorsiflexed so that it touches the anterior shin without any deviation, and this excluded club foot.

Great care should be taken to rule out spina bifida and poliomyelitis.

Varying degrees of club foot may be considered in cerebral palsy and arthrogryposis.

Prognosis

Without treatment, the deformity increases, the gait becomes unsightly due to troublesome painful corns and callosities.

With early, effective, and continued treatment, all cases of club foot can be cured and a useful properly shaped foot can be obtained.

In the other children, the condition can be greatly improved.

Treatment

The main object of treatment is mainly two, namely,

1. To correct the deformity
2. Develop the muscle power to such an extent to maintain the correction

The most important aspect of forefoot deformity is that the corrected forefoot points 20° outward. Following this, the hindfoot must be brought into a vertical plane before the equinus can be corrected.

Treatment of an Early Case

The treatment should begin as early as possible when the child is born.

Manipulation: This treatment can be repeated at regular intervals.
Splintage and plaster immobilization: Following manipulation, some form of a splint is used.

A Dennis Brown splint allows full correction of the deformity, although allowing activity which is very important from the muscular development point of view. This treatment can be continued for about 9 months of age.

A complication that one must be careful of is a rocker-bottom foot, which is produced by over-correction of the fixed equinus deformity. It becomes apparent after a period of time that the equinus deformity has not been corrected fully when it becomes necessary to consider a subcutaneous tenotomy of the tendocalcaneus. Occasionally the plantar fascia also requires to be divided. Following these procedures, a above knee POP cast is required for 4 weeks in an over-corrected position with the knee in flexion and the leg in external rotation.

Treatment of Old and Relapsed Cases

In a small percentage of cases, because of rigidity and a constant tendency to relapse, the manipulation treatment is not sufficient, then a plantigrade foot can be obtained by soft tissue release, mainly on the medial side along with tendocalcaneus length-ening with or without a posterior capsulotomy.

Treatment in the Adult Patient

In an adult patient, no manipulation or soft tissue release will be helpful in correct-ing the deformity and a cuneiform tarsectomy is the most reliable method than an osteotomy.

In other cases, a Naughton-Dunn's triple arthrodesis may be considered when the mid-tarsal and sub-taloid joints are arthrodesed.

Other Forms of Club Foot

1. *Muscular type*: A type of club foot may be seen in a rare congenital affection of the legs and arms, known as arthrogryposis multiplex congenita. Here the foot deformity is extreme and is more rigid than the ordinary type. There is usually a fixed flexion deformity of the knees and hips.
2. *The osseous type*: Here the club foot is associated with partial or complete absence of the tibia, and this may be associated with other abnormalities such as absence of toes or failure of development of the bones of the tarsus.

Painful Conditions of the Ankle

Sprains of the Ankle Joint

This usually results from a twisting injury resulting in damage to the deltoid and lateral collateral ligaments of the ankle. They can be graded as mild, moderate, and severe, depending on the amount of fibers torn, giving rise to varying degrees of ankle instability. Examination reveals there is a swelling, bruising, and local tenderness over the affected ligaments. Radiographs are essential to distinguish ligamentous injury to fractures of the lateral malleolus, showing a talar shift, indicating a strong inversion injury and above all stress radiographs are very helpful.

The talotibial joint is a hinge joint with dorsiflexion and plantar flexion, along with minimal rotation, particularly accompanying the tibiocalcaneal movements. The stress tests are ideally compared with both ankles together when they show an average tilt of 3–27°, which is increased in ligamentous injuries of the ankle.

Treatment in mild cases is to support the damaged ligament by a pad and bandaging with a local injection of hydrocortisone along with graduated ankle exercises. A moderate injury requires immobilization in a plaster cast for 3 weeks before starting with graduated exercises. In severe cases or complete rupture of the ligaments, this immobilization may be carried on for 6–10 weeks before starting with graduated exercises. Failure to treat sprains may result in the syndrome of chronic strain when the patient keeps falling over along with pain and swelling. Radiographs are very helpful in showing a talar tilt to rule out a complete rupture of the ligament.

Treatment is mainly aimed at preventing the twisting episodes by lowering the heel and flaring out the lateral edge of the heel by 6 mm. The actual episode is treated by an injection of a local anesthetic or hydrocortisone injections along with bandaging.

Traumatic Arthritis of the Ankle

This is often called as the "footballer's ankle," as it is seen most commonly in athletes. Here there is definite history of a twisting injury followed by generalized dull aching pain along with tenderness in the affected area. Radiographs are negative and an effusion may be seen in some cases.

Treatment mainly consists of resting sport, a supporting bandage along with graduated physiotherapy before allowing to return to sport. Repeated minor trauma to the capsular attachment and repeated compression injuries of the bones which are in contact during extreme dorsi- and plantar flexion may result in the production of small bone exostoses in the tibial margin and malleoli and on the neck of the talus. In cases of effusion, immobilization may be for 3 weeks as necessary. If conservative treatment fails, then operation can be considered to remove the bony outgrowths and immobilization may be for 4 weeks thereafter.

Rupture of the Tendocalcaneus

This condition usually results in middle life in badminton or tennis players. The rupture is usually complete with a feeling of giving way in the narrowest part of the tendon about 4 cm above the insertion. The line of rupture may be transverse and clean like an incised wound or ragged from the projecting bundles of tendon fibers. The sheath may or may not remain intact and is rapidly filled with blood and its walls become edematous. The plantaris usually escapes damage. Incomplete ruptures are very rare, except at the musculotendinous junction, and this is usually diagnosed by ultrasonography when usually they are left alone because they heal well on their own without need for any surgery.

Clinical Features

At the moment of rupture, the patient may experience sharp pain when there is immediate disability and when in a short while swelling and tenderness appear. Even the patient may be able to walk without experiencing severe pain.

In treated cases, the sheath may become adherent to the retracted ends of the tendon and may act as a feeble bond of union, thus enabling a certain amount of muscular contraction to occur. The calf muscles are shortened and there may be a permanent decrease of plantar-flexion.

Diagnosis

When the rupture is within 24–48 h when seen, the examination is rendered difficult by the edema. The following points enable to diagnose the condition.

1. The presence of a gap which accommodates the examining finger and which is increased by dorsiflexion of the foot.
2. Unduely high level of the prominences caused by the bellies of the calf muscles.
3. An abnormal range of passive dorsiflexion compared with the normal opposite side. This sign is absent in cases of partial rupture.
4. Inability to perform or marked limitation of plantar-flexion.

A very specific test depending on the continuity of the gastrocnemius soleus-calcaneus complex is known as Thompson's test. When the mass of the calf is compressed by hand with the patient lying in the prone position, and the foot being free at the end of the table, plantar-flexion of the ankle does occur passively. However, when there is a complete rupture of the tendocalcaneus, there is no movement at the foot.

Differential diagnosis consists of a ruptured popliteal Baker's cyst into the calf which sometimes occurs in rheumatoid patients or a localized thrombophlebitis of the short saphenous vein must also be excluded.

Treatment

A recent complete rupture must always be repaired as soon as possible, with the ankle plantar-flexed and the knee flexed to relax the calf when the ends are repaired with silk sutures (Fig. 12.4).

When the ends are ragged, the ends are freshened and the repair is augmented by fasica lata, and wherever possible the sheath is also carefully repaired. After the

Fig. 12.4 Rupture of the
tendo-achillis (Courtesy:
Dilip Malhotra, Bahrain)

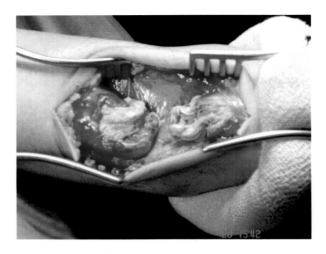

operation, the leg is immobilized in an above knee plaster cast with the ankle in complete plantar-flexion and the knee flexed to 30°. After 3 weeks, the foot is gently brought to the neutral position of right angle and the plaster re-applied, and the patient is allowed to walk. In 6 weeks, the plaster is removed entirely gently and the patient allowed to walk in a shoe with an elevated heel. Massage, faradism, and exercises in walking may all be used in this convalescence period.

Operative repair is also advised in old neglected ruptures associated with instability of the leg. Various techniques are used to repair this defect. The best method is to turn down superficial strips from the broad part and the superficial surface of both the parts exposed with their surfaces cleared of fibrous tissue when the length of the strips are long enough to reach the ruptured site. These strips are drawn through in opposite directions with the foot in plantar-flexion, and drawn taut and fixed with the tendon with silk. Post-operatively a below knee plaster with the foot held in equinus to relax the tension on the suture line is applied for 4–6 weeks.

Rupture of the Plantaris Tendon

This condition results in minimum disability and conservative treatment usually gives good results.

The patient sits on a table and allows his foot to hang at its edge. Several pieces of adhesive plaster are made to encircle the thickest part of the calf. Then an elastoplast bandage is applied from the foot to below the knee. By this means, pain is relieved and healing encouraged.

In certain cases, slight elevation of the heel of the boot is able to cure this condition.

Fusion of the Ankle Joint

This is indicated when there are significant symptoms from asymmetrical joint surfaces along with severe pain, swelling with instability and limitation of movement.

Such a clinical situation may arise from any disease or deformity, such as infection, tuberculosis, or trauma such as a Pott's fracture dislocation and osteochondritis.

The position of the foot is extremely vital to this procedure to achieve a satisfactory walking gait. In a person if the ankle joint is fixed at 90° and there is no other leg or foot deformity, the individual can walk without any limp, especially if there is mid-tarsal mobility. A plantigrade position of the foot must be achieved. In a woman, the position of 100° is acceptable to accommodate the height of the heel.

Arthrodesis of the Ankle Joint

Since some torsional movement of the foot occurs within the plaster, it is preferable to cut a graft from the distal end of the tibia, turn it upside down, and then drive it to be firmly wedged into the slot prepared in the talus.

An alternative acceptable method is Charnley's compression arthrodesis by applying compression through clamps with a pin inserted through the distal tibia and the calcaneus, and with excision of the articular surfaces. This method reduces the time of immobilization with a plaster cast giving good results.

Disturbances of the Peroneal Tendons

Peroneal Palsy due to Hematoma

Peroneal palsy due to hematoma in the common peroneal nerve has been known after distal tibial fractures and inversion ankle sprains.

Persistent pain, numbness, and severe pain with any motion may not occur for hours or even days after the injury and may not be readily connected with the peroneal nerve in the presence of injury to the distal leg. Awareness of the vulnerability of the vasa nervorum of the common peroneal nerve helps to determine the level of exploration.

Examination for a hematoma at the level of swelling and tenderness along the common peroneal nerve below the sciatic bifurcation and the possibility of the hematoma shutting off the blood supply of the nerve should always be kept in mind.

Foot Drop in Leprosy

Paralysis of the dorsiflexors, namely, the tibialis anterior and the extensors and evertors, namely, the peronei, is a very common feature which is disabling in leprosy. However, the high prevalence of infection, secondary contractures, mainly involving the tendo-calcaneus, and difficulty in balancing a foot due to tendon lengthening along with instability of the talonavicular joint with dropping of the toes have been described. Recently, splitting of the distal end of the tibialis posterior into two halves and insertion of a half into the extensor hallucis longus and the other into the extensor digitorum and peroneus brevis more laterally with the ankle held in 10 degrees of dorsiflexion and the knee in 30 degrees of flexion. The tendocalcaneus is lengthened by a Z-plasty if contracture is present. This is immobilized in a plaster cast which is removed at 6 weeks when walking is permitted.

Tenosynovitis

As in DeQuervain's stenosing tenosynovitis at the wrist, anatomical anomalies can occur in the tendon masses of the posterior tibial compartment.

There is pain, swelling, and local tenderness with occasional crepitus proximal to the calcaneal tubercle, but below and behind the lateral malleolus. Resisted eversion movement will aggravate the pain in these cases.

Treatment is by physiotherapy, short wave diathermy, and some form of partial immobilization, injections of hydrocortisone is also helpful in some cases and partial or total excision of the tendon sheath may be considered in some cases.

Dislocation of the Peroneal Tendons

Dislocation of the peroneal tendons upward and forward from their normal position behind the lateral malleolus is not rare at all and this may affect one or both tendons. This condition usually occurs in children and a snap is also felt at the time of dislocation.

The lesion is traumatic or can also result from congenital malformation of the groove in which the tendons lie. In paralytic talipes calcaneo-valgus, a similar displacement may be occasionally seen. The displacement usually occurs when the foot is dorsiflexed and abducted.

The signs include local swelling and ecchymosis. The function of the foot is not seriously impaired when the patient feels that something has given way in the foot or the tendons may be found to lie anterior to the lateral malleolus.

A recurrent dislocation is not infrequently seen in these cases.

Treatment

In recent cases, the tendons should be kept in place by an adhesive plaster applied over a felt pad kept over and behind the lateral malleolus.

In recurrent cases, the groove behind and below the lateral malleolus is deepened by means of a sliding graft of bone from the lateral malleolus.

An alternative to this is when a strip of the tendocalcaneus is threaded through the fibula and attached on to itself, thereby making it function like a retinaculum.

Chapter 13
The Great Toe

K. Mohan Iyer

Affection of the Bones and Joints of the Metatarsus

The Normal Form of the Forefoot

The metatarsal bones are normally arranged as a parallel series, with the first metatarsal being thicker and stronger than the others, thereby providing a weight-bearing foot. Furthermore, it becomes the fulcrum on which the body weight is swung forward during walking, with its head lying more in an anterior plane than the others. The other important weight-bearing points are the fifth metatarsal and the calcaneus, and these with the first metatarsal head are regarded as the three points of the tripod.

The intermediate metatarsal heads are sometimes said to form the anterior metatarsal arch.

Developmental Anomalies of the Metatarsus

During the course of development, the first metatarsal is gradually drawn laterally from the abducted position parallel to its neighbors when it loses its mobility and grows in strength till it overstrips its fellows. The common developmental errors are as follows:

1. *Metatarsus primus varus*: In this condition, the first metatarsal is distinctly abducted from the midline of the second and there is a palpable and radiological interval, which is sometimes occupied by an accessory ossicle called the Os inter-metatarseum (Fig. 13.1).

K.M. Iyer
Consultant Orthopedic Surgeon, Bangalore University,
152, Kailash Apartments 8th Main, Malleswaram 120/H-2K,
560 003 Bangalore, Karnataka, India
e-mail: kmiyer28@hotmail.com

K.M. Iyer (ed.), *Orthopedics of the Upper and Lower Limb*,
DOI 10.1007/978-1-4471-4447-2_13, © Springer-Verlag London 2013

Fig. 13.1 Os Inter-metatarseum (Courtesy: Magdi
E. Greiss, Whitehaven, Cumbria, UK)

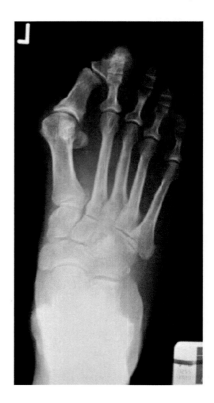

2. *Metatarsus atavicus or brevis*: In this condition, the metatarsus is shorter than
   normal and its metatarsal head is situated behind the head of the second and commonly the third. The metatarsal is often abducted (primus varus).
3. *Metatarsus hypermobilicus*: In this condition, the first metatarsal is unduly
   mobile.

Clinical Effect of Developmental Anomalies

In the metatarsus primus varus, the first metatarsal is lying away from the long axis
of the foot and hence fails to act as an effective fulcrum, its function therefore is
assumed by the second metatarsal and possibly the third metatarsal.
In metatarsal atavicus a similar effect is there.

In metatarsus hypermobilicus, the first metatarsal though it may act as a fulcrum
very effectively, though it is fixed by the adductor muscle, and without such fixation
fails to function as a stable weight-bearing point of the tripod and hence becomes
splayed out on long standing.

There is one important function of the effect of metatarsus primus varus when
even the cause of ordinary footwear will cause the toe to get displaced. The increased

load thrown on the intermediate metatarsal heads is a factor underlying a series of interesting and important disturbances, namely,

1. Hallux valgus
2. Metatarsalgia
3. March foot or March fracture
4. Kohler's disease of the metatarsal head or Freiberg's infraction

Hallux Valgus

The deformity of hallux valgus consists of adduction of the proximal phalanyx of the great toe toward the midline of the foot along with varying degrees of varus of the first metatarsal (Figs. 13.2 and 13.3).

This phalangeal deviation is further increased by contracture and shortening of the adductor hallucis and extensor hallucis longus, so much so that the base of the first phalanx is displaced so far laterally that it articulates with only the lateral condyle metatarsal head, leaving the medial condyle of the metatarsal as a prominence on the medial side of the foot, which is subjected to friction and pressure from the shoe. An adventitious bursa forms over it and the projecting bone along with its bursa and corn or callosity is collectively known as a bunion (Fig. 13.4).

Pathology

The tissues on the lateral side of the deformity, namely, the capsule, muscle tendons, and ligaments are adaptively shortened while the capsule and ligaments on the medial side are stretched. The cartilage on the exposed part of the head of the metatarsal undergoes fibrillation and degeneration along with marginal osteophytes as in osteoarthritis. The function of the intrinsic muscles of the foot are affected to be known as anterior metatarsalgia. A secondary feature is the development of hammer toe along with dorsiflexion of the proximal phalanx and in some cases even complete subluxation of the second metatarsophalangeal joint.

Clinical Features

Many people suffer from very little symptoms till later on it is mainly pain due to arthritis when the bursa may become enlarged or even suppurate.

When symptoms are due to arthritis, the range of movements in the affected joint are reduced and painful.

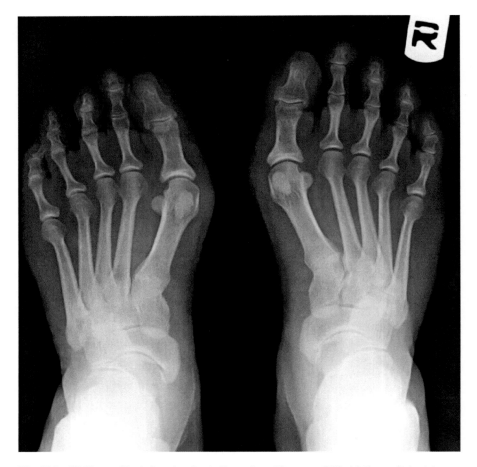

Fig. 13.2 AP X-ray of both feet showing hallux valgus (Courtesy: Dilip Malhotra, Bahrain)

The pain from hallux valgus may be due to one of the following causes:

1. Friction and pressure over the prominent head with production of bursitis.
2. Osteoarthritis of the joint.
3. Involvement of the sesamoid bones in the arthritis process.
4. Callosities beneath the second and third metatarsal heads due to splaying of the transverse arch.

Treatment

Conservative Treatment

Initial treatment can be by the provision of special shoes with a raised inner side along with a metatarsal bar beneath the metatarsal heads.

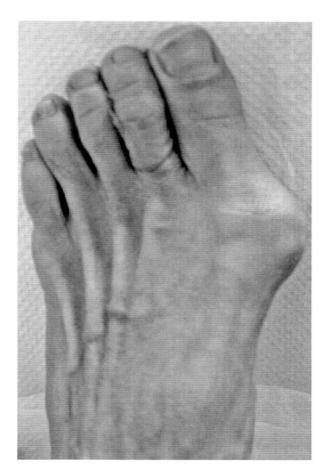

Fig. 13.3 Clinical photograph showing hallux valgus with a bunion (Courtesy: Dilip Malhotra, Bahrain) (Reproduced with kind permission of Springer Verlag)

Operative Treatment

This is mainly carried out for the relief of pain:

(a) Conservative operation involving removal of the exostosis and bursa.
(b) *Keller's operation*: This is done in a majority of cases and it involves excision of the proximal two-thirds of the phalanx, care being taken to avoid injury to the flexor tendon.
(c) *Scarf osteotomy*: This is the generally accepted form of diaphyseal osteotomy, which is performed in various centers and it has an effect of removing pressure on the bunion also, giving good results (Fig. 13.5).
(d) *Arthrodesis of the first metatarsophalangeal joint*: This mainly aims at preserving the strength and function of the great toe.
(e) *McBride operation*: In this procedure, the lateral deforming force of the conjoined tendons of the adductor hallucis along with the lateral head of the flexor hallucis brevis is transferred from the proximal phalanx to the lateral side of the

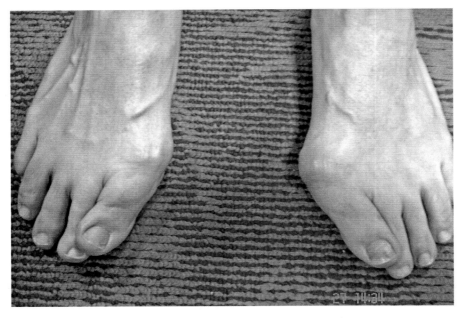

Fig. 13.4 Bilateral hallux valgus (Courtesy: Dilip Malhotra, Bahrain)

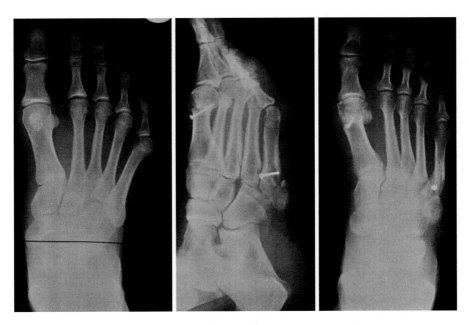

Fig. 13.5 Treated by a reverse scarf osteotomy (Courtesy: Magdi E. Greiss, Whitehaven, Cumbria, UK)

head of the first metatarsal. The lateral sesamoid and the exostosis are also removed to obtain normal alignment of the hallux.

(f) *Radical type of operation*: This operation mainly aims at (1) correction of the deformity, (2) maintenances of correction, and (3) restoration of muscle balance. Here the exostosis along with the proximal third of the proximal phalanx is removed and the adducted metatarsal is corrected by an osteotomy at its base, which is maintained by insertion of a graft and the attachment of the adductor hallucis is transferred to the metatarsal head to give it stability.

(g) *Osteotomy-bunionectomy*: This is conventionally known as Mitchel's operation when the hallux is displaced laterally after removal of the exostosis.

(h) A McBride Bunion type operation is very useful for adolescents and young adults. Here a wedge osteotomy is done at the base of the first metatarsal along removal of the lateral sesamoid and the adductor hallucis tendon is then transferred to the head of the first metatarsal.

Hallux Rigidus

It is a condition of stiffness of the great toe when the dorsiflexion of the great toe is absent. In the early cases when the plantar flexion is present, it is called as hallux flexus.

Rigidity (Fig. 13.6) may be associated with inflammatory changes such as rheumatism or from a traumatic lesion, giving rise to muscular spasm.

In the static variety of hallux rigidus, there may be concomitant flat foot. In both varieties, the rigid joint in the later stages becomes the seat of osteoarthritis.

Clinical Features

Here the main symptom is pain which is experienced on walking and more so at the take-off stage of gait. The joint is sometimes swollen due to periarthritis along with several marginal osteophytes at the dorsal edge of the articular surface of the metatarsal head.

Treatment

Conservative Treatment

Relief may be obtained by (a) thickening of the sole of the shoe, (b) by insertion of a thin plate of tempered steel between both layers of the sole, or (c) by fitting a metatarsal bar to the shoe.

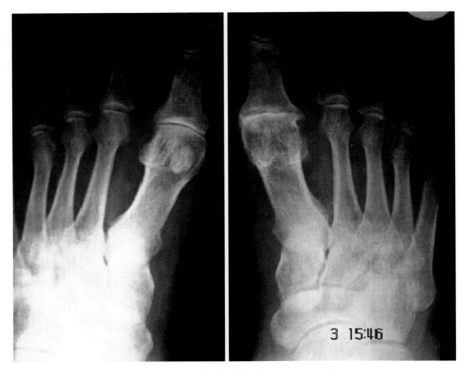

Fig. 13.6 Anteroposterior radiograph of both feet showing hallux rigidus of the right great toe (Courtesy: Dilip Malhotra, Bahrain) (Reproduced with kind permission of Springer Verlag)

In certain cases with a short history, overcorrection of the deformity along with application of a walking plaster cast which is retained for 4–6 weeks may be helpful.

Operative Treatment

Majority of the cases are treated by a Keller's procedure or by arthrodesis of the metatarsophalangeal joint.

Hallux Flexus

This is usually a static deformity that occurs during walking which may become fixed and rigid. Here there is a marked plantar flexion of the proximal phalanx of the big toe along with some degree of dorsiflexion of the first metatarsal. Soft tissue contractures occur in the capsule and particularly the flexor hallucis longus and brevis tendons, resulting in loss of mobility of the first metatarsophalangeal joint.

This condition may be seen in:

1. Poliomyelitis in which there is paralysis of all the foot muscles, except gastrone-mius along with normal flexors of the toes, as well as flexor hallucis brevis.
2. Certain tendon transfer operations in which there is a failure to obtain a balance between the peroneus longus and the tibialis anterior muscle.
3. The onset of arthritic hallux rigidus resulting in a soft tissue contracture, involving the plantar structures.
4. A rocker-bottom deformity of a vertical talus or congenital flat foot.

Walking is difficult because of pain and also because of inversion deformity of the forefoot.

Treatment is by means of a Lapidus procedure, in which the insertion of the tibialis anterior is transferred backward to the insertion of the tendon of the tibialis posterior or at the navicular tubercle. A wedge osteotomy may be carried out at the naviculo-cuneiform-metatarsal joints, and the flexor hallucis longus tendon is divided at its insertion and transferred proximally through an oblique drill hole in the shaft of the first metatarsal to become a plantar flexor of the first metatarsal. These may be coupled with plantar capsulotomies along with excision of the dorsal bunion.

Metatarsalgia

It is pain beneath the metatarsal heads or shafts of the metatarsals and is of three varieties: (1) Traumatic, (2) inflammatory, or (3) static.

The static variety is frequently found in association with developmental anomalies particularly metatarsus primus varus and metatarsus hypermobilis or a debilitating illness when the foot muscles are atonic.

When the interosseous muscles contract, they flex the metatarsophalangeal joints, extend the toe joints and bring the metatarsal heads together. Failure of these muscles permits splaying of the foot and curling of the toes. The extra weight is borne by the metatarsal heads with a strain on the longitudinal arch ligament and this type of metatarsalgia is called relaxation metatarsalgia.

When the metatarsal heads are crowded together, such as may occur from wearing narrow shoes, the digital nerve that passes between them may be compressed or irritated and this may produce neuritis to be called as compression metatarsalgia or Morton's metatarsalgia.

In addition to these, metatarsal pain may be seen in Kohler's disease and march foot.

Clinical Features

In the first static or ligamentous type, the pain is just beneath the metatarsal heads, which is relieved by lateral compression of the metatarsal heads.

The foot is broader than normal, the splay type and there are obvious deficiencies between the metatarsal heads due to atrophy of the interossei muscles. The clawing of the toes that occurs is mainly because of involvement of lumbricals and interossei when the proximal phalanges get dorsiflexed along with callosities beneath the metatarsal heads.

Morton's Metatarsalgia

In this neuritic type of foot, the forefoot appears compressed. It may affect any digital nerves but the most common is the nerve in relation to the third or fourth metatarsal space.

Parasthesiae with actual sensory loss may be present.

Pain is reproduced by dorsoplantar compression of the metatarsal space at the level of the metatarsal heads.

The cause of the neuromatous formation is unknown but may be due to local irritation or obstruction.

Some people think it is due to an endarteritis obliterans of the accompanying metatarsal artery while some people think it is due to bulging of the intermetatarsal bursa along with stretching of the dorsal communicating artery.

Treatment

The main aim of treatment is to strength the muscles that support the forefoot and to keep the forefoot in a corrected position till the intrinsic muscles are strengthened by exercises and re-education.

Support

1. In all types, fitting of a specially designed shoe is advisable, which should have a straight inner side, a broad thick sole, a low heel and a metatarsal bar or crescent well behind the heads of the metatarsals.
2. In more severe cases, the support must be applied directly to the foot and this may be carried out by a felt pad and adhesive strapping which is changed at intervals of a week.
3. In some cases, some permanent means of supporting the anterior arch is necessary, such as a thick leather insole.

Operation

In most cases, resection of the head and neck of the affected metatarsals will suffice.

When the clinical diagnosis suggests a neuroma of the digital nerve, it is explored by a web splitting incision and dissection is carried out till the neuroma is identified, which is completely excised. The neuroma may also be approached by a plantar incision. Walking is allowed after an interval of 3 weeks with supports.

March Foot or March Fracture

This was seen as a developmental anomaly consisting of subperiosteal deposits of osteoid tissue on the shafts of one or other of the second, third, and fourth metatarsal bones.

Clinical Features

This condition is most commonly seen in the second metatarsal but may occur in the third or fourth metatarsal and is not infrequently bilateral.

The condition may begin insidiously with a puffy edema of the forefoot when the foot is subjected to abnormal use such as in long marching. Sometimes there may be pain right from the start.

Radiographic examination of the foot repeatedly may show a fusiform swelling around the neck of the metatarsal.

Etiology

It is clinically and radiological similar to stress fractures that occur in the tibia and other weight-bearing bones.

Some people believe that it is caused by spasm of the interossei muscles through which the vessels entering and leaving the bone penetrate, leading to vascular obstruction and consequent edema of the soft tissues and periosteum, with the periosteum being thick and spongy and the edema resulting in rarefaction of the bone, thus rendering it brittle.

Some believe that the primary factor is a developmental anomaly leading to mechanical insufficiency of the first metatarsal. Here the second metatarsal must assume the role of the first metatarsal in providing for take-off during walking, and this foot is structurally weak when a slight trauma results in a fracture.

Treatment

When indicated in the acute stage, immobilization in a plaster cast for 4–6 weeks will give immense relief.

In cases seen at a late stage with minimal symptoms, the application of a metatarsal bar to the sole of the foot should be adequate for relief. Pain disappears on healing with thickening of the metatarsal.

Freiberg's Infraction

It is a condition where the metatarsal head is broadened, usually the second and less often the third and then the others. Clinically there is pain and stiffness at the metatarsophalangeal joint.

Pathology

The earliest change is slight subperiosteal osteoporosis, with the porotic area being situated in the dorsal part of the articular surface. This porotic area increases in size, along with indentation and collapse of the articular surface. Later this area becomes sequestrated to lie finally in the joint as a loose body.

Etiology

This condition is very similar to other epiphyseal lesions such as Perthes' and Osgood-Schlatter's disease. Here the primary condition is either a traumatic fracture or infraction of the articular surface similar to osteochondritis dessicans.

There is often considerable thickening of the metatarsal shaft which is a compensatory phenomenon to strengthen the second metatarsal (Fig. 13.7).

Clinical Features

This condition may occur at any age before the epiphysis is fused.
    The radiologic changes are as follows:

1. Broadening of the metatarsal head
2. The head is irregular in contour and flat
3. The joint space is increased
4. The shaft of the metatarsal is thick
5. Detached portion of the articular surface may lie free in the joint

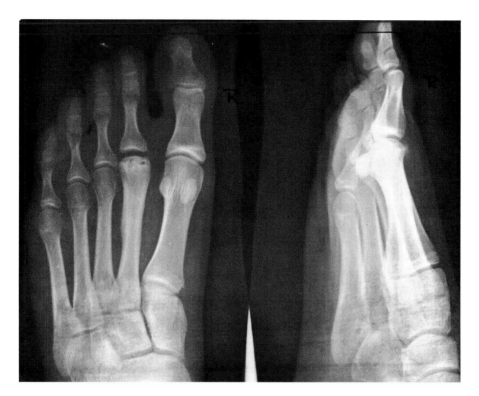

Fig. 13.7 Freiberg's infraction (Courtesy: Magdi E. Greiss, Whitehaven, Cumbria, UK)

Treatment

In acute stage, a below knee walking plaster may give relief.

In mild cases, the use of a metatarsal bar or pad may be necessary.

In refractory cases, relief is obtained by excision of the head of the metatarsal, though it may lead to weakening of the transverse arch.

Ingrowing Toe Nail (Onycho-cryptosis)

This is a very painful condition and is caused mainly by the pressure against the shoe, with the soft tissues being forced against the nail. The pain is caused by the splinter of nail growing forward along the lateral groove into the soft tissues. This lateral edge of the nail which is mainly hidden is not adequately cut when it grows forward and penetrates the subcutaneous tissues, often carrying infection with it.

Treatment

Prophylaxis

The nail should be cut at right angles to its long axis and not convexly, which destroys to some extent the protective infolding of its edge.

Conservation Treatment

This mainly consists of removing all possible sources of infection such as narrow shoes or stockings and in removing the irritation caused by the pressure of the nail edge.

Operative Treatment

This should not be carried out in the presence of acute infection.

This is known as Zadek's procedure and it consists in radical removal of the sharp edge of the nail along with its underlying matrix, when a V-shaped wedge, including about a third of the breadth of the nail along with the nail fold, is excised from the lateral surface of the nail. The edges cannot be brought together and most of the wound is allowed to granulate.

This operation is not always successful as spicules of the nail grow out at its edges giving rise to pain. Amputation of the tip of the toe with removal of the nail bed often gives a good result without affecting function.

Suture must be avoided in the presence of chronic sepsis, and a small Vaseline dressing must be applied to the raw area which is left to heal by granulation tissue. Excessive reduction of granulation tissue can be achieved by repeated application of copper sulphate crystals.

Subungual Hematoma

This usually occurs when the toe is tramped upon and is seen as a minute reddish-black speck which is visible under the nail, but in some cases the entire nail may become black from effused blood when the nail may be shed if untreated.

This hemorrhage may result in a considerable lot of pain and considerable relief may be obtained by drilling or trephining the nail over the blood with a large needle. Recurrence can be prevented by applying a pressure bandage for 24 h along with a digital nerve local anesthetic.

Onycho-gryposis

This condition is also called as a ram's horn nail and it usually affects the great toe with hypertrophy of the nail, which is irregular and hard, cross ridged and is curved upward.

Treatment

The ideal treatment is complete excision of the nail bed or an amputation of the terminal phalynx.

Subungual Exostosis

This is usually due to old injuries or due to a recent injury when due to a mild periostitis there is a cartilaginous outgrowth beneath the nail which becomes osseous.

This is frequently seen in women around the ages of 12–30 years.

The main complaint is pain which is worse on wearing a shoe and X-rays are diagnostic.

The ideal method of treatment is complete excision of the nail and the operated site may be painted with phenol followed by alcohol, with a tulle gras dressing applied over it with pressure.

The Sesamoid Bones of the Great Toe

The cartilaginous precursors of the sesamoid bones appear in early fetal life, but do not ossify till between the ages of 8 and 11. This ossification usually occurs from a single center, but very occasionally may be from multiple centers which then fuse to a single center. In 10 % of individuals, these centers do not unite resulting in a multipartite sesamoid.

Fracture of the sesamoid bones

The sesamoid bones of the great toe, particularly the medial one, are occasionally fractured. The violence may be direct or indirect, either by falls or heavy objects falling on the toe.

The main symptoms are pain, which is situated over the affected sesamoid and is affected by movement of the metatarsophalangeal joint of the great toe. Tenderness is usually elicited by plantar pressure over the affected sesamoid.

The diagnosis is made with considerable caution on radiographs due to the frequency of the multipartite condition.

The treatment is by a plaster-of-paris cast which includes the great toe for 3–6 weeks. If this treatment is not satisfactory, then careful excision of the affected sesamoid bone is advised.

Overlapping of the Fifth Toe

This is a frequent congenital lesion due to constriction of the tissues on the dorsum of the toe, which draws into a varus position along with subluxation.

It is mainly a congenital deformity in 50 % of the cases and presents with difficulty in wearing shoes.

Treatment of this condition ranges from a V-Y plasty to amputation, but the most widely accepted operation is a Butler's operation when through a dorsal racquet incision the extensor tendon with the dorsal capsule of the metatarsophalangeal joint is divided with the adherent plantar capsule being stripped off the metatarsal head and the skin closed.

Hammer Toe

This is a deformity that consists of dorsiflexion of the proximal phalanyx, plantar flexion of the second, and flexion or extension of the distal phalanyx. It usually affects the second toe and is usually bilateral, and is most commonly caused by overcrowding of the toes due to ill-fitting shoes. It is also commonly associated with hallux valgus with the displacement of the great toe forcing the second toe which is longer into a flexed position (Fig. 13.8). This condition usually begins in childhood and the patient usually complains of a painful corn and bunion.

It is mainly treated by a reduction of the contracted ligaments. In young children, repeated manipulation is carried out holding the corrected position by strips of adhesive plaster passing over and under the affected toe with its neighbors.

In adults, an operation is usually indicated and two types of operation are carried out as follows:

1. With a semilunar incision made transversely over the dorsum of the affected joint, the corn and bursa is excised and a "spike" operation is done with the head of the proximal phalanx nibbled like a spike and then inserted into a hole in the base of the middle phalanyx correcting the deformity.

Fig. 13.8 Clinical
photograph showing hammer
toes. The *arrow* in the
photograph indicates the side
to be operated (*right side*)
(Courtesy: Dilip Malhotra,
Bahrain) (Reproduced with
kind permission of Springer
Verlag)

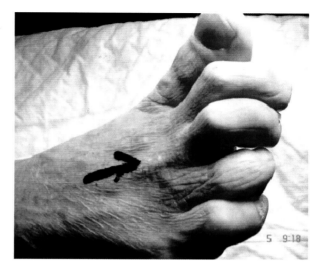

2. Another type of fusion of the interphalangeal joint is done by clearing out the articular surfaces and transfixing it with a K wire by holding it in a reduced position.

In both these operations, it is necessary to carry out a tenotomy of the structures on the dorsum of the metatarsophalangeal joint to ensure correction of the dorsiflexion of the proximal joint.

Kohler's Disease of the Tarsal Navicular

Unfortunately two quite different conditions have been named as Kohler's disease, one affecting the navicular bone in the foot and the other one being the head of the second metatarsal, which is also called Freiberg's infraction.

Kohler's disease of the tarsal navicular affects boys more than girls. The disease is very similar to an osteochondritis, whose cause is yet unknown.

Clinically there is pain and swelling in the region of the tarsal navicular, and there is tenderness on pressure which is increased on weight-bearing.

Radiographs are very helpful in showing definite narrowing of the bone in its anteroposterior diameter, along with a condensation of the bony structure. There is no fragmentation of the bony nucleus (Fig. 13.9).

The navicular is the last bone in the foot to ossify and it forms the keystone of the longitudinal arch, which is subjected to a lot of strain while in a cartilaginous state. It can ossify from two or three separate multiple centers, thus giving the appearance of irregular ossification. The diagnosis of circulatory interference is definite when there is a true loss of expected transverse diameter along with increased density of the bone.

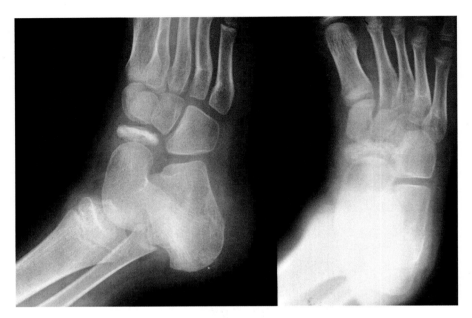

Fig. 13.9 Kohler's disease of the tarsal navicular (Courtesy: Magdi E. Greiss, Whitehaven, Cumbria, UK)

Treatment

Usually symptomatic recovery occurs in a few months and if painful, below knee plaster cast is helpful with non-weight-bearing being on crutches. This can be later on followed by foot exercises, gentle massage, and contrast baths to the affected foot.

Index

K.M. Iyer (ed.), *Orthopedics of the Upper and Lower Limb*,
DOI 10.1007/978-1-4471-4447-2, © Springer-Verlag London 2013

Printed by Publishers' Graphics LLC
CIMO20121005.19.18.11